Be Good to Your Body

Be Good to Your Body

by TRENT BUSBY, A.B., M.D., F.A.C.S.
Diplomate American Board Obstetrics and Gynecology

The Citadel Press Secaucus, N.J.

Second printing, 1977

Published by Citadel Press
A division of Lyle Stuart, Inc.
120 Enterprise Ave., Secaucus, N. J. 07094
In Canada: George J. McLeod Limited
73 Bathurst St., Toronto, Ont.
Manufactured in the United States of America
ISBN 0-8065-0558-3

LIBRARY OF CONGRESS CATALOGING IN PUBLICATION DATA
Busby, Trent.
Be good to your body.
1. Women—Health and hygiene. 2. Women—Diseases.
3. Hygiene, Sexual. I. Title.
RG121.B92 613.9'54 76-41759
ISBN 0-8065-0558-3

To my wife and children,
who generally agree with,
but don't always follow,
my advice

Contents

Preface

The old saw, "If you put your hand in the fire, it will burn," originated years ago, when fire was one of man's greatest dangers. In our modern, highly technical, supersophisticated society, this saying should be extended in depth and breadth to say, "Don't do anything dumb." Lurking innocently in stores and markets all around us are potentially dangerous and hazardous products hawked by all the media, many of which have already been exposed by numerous books, newspapers, and magazine articles. The most gullible victims are women—particularly young women. Perhaps they are more infatuated by the miracle of the boob tube than the articles advertised thereon. To me it is incredible that anyone can suffer through the commercials on eye makeup, detergents, toilet paper, douches, and hair preparations without being overcome with disgust.

My purpose is to discuss multiple facets of female health and hygiene, especially as they pertain to sexuality. The busy physician of today, although he may know these things, will seldom take the time to tell his patients of these hazards, and some physicians are not even aware of many of the problems I am going to mention. As a matter of fact, a recent medical survey indicates that three-fourths of physicians—including gynecologists—are unqualified for, and uncomfortable with discussing sexual problems with patients! Although I am not a women's liberationist, it is obvious in many respects that this movement has done much to enlighten women about the care and appreciation of their bodies and their right to sexual fulfillment.

When I was a medical student at Johns Hopkins some thirty years ago, it was one of the few medical schools in the United States that required psychiatry classes for four years. During this time only one hour was devoted to sex and that dealt only with perversions. As to everyday hygiene and common sense, there is no such course offered in any medical school. What little I know about this subject has been gathered from my practice, talking with people of all ages, reading all sorts of scientific, pornographic, and fallacious material, and applying a modicum of reasonable judgment in separating the wheat from the chaff.

The information herein presented has been gleaned from twenty-five years of practicing gynecology and perusing the medical literature of this era. Various, seemingly unrelated subjects will be presented, mainly because over the years I have admittedly developed certain pet peeves and strong feelings in certain areas which I would like to share with you. This book is not a gospel; it only represents the opinions of the author. On the other hand, most women will find some enlightenment in it which may give them better physical and mental health. As I have told many patients, only my fee is mandatory—the advice, optional.

TRENT BUSBY

Salisbury, North Carolina

Be Good to Your Body

CHAPTER 1

Wrappers

SINCE Adam's fig leaf, it has been customary for people to wear clothes, particularly to cover the genitalia. Although originally clothing was to provide modesty and warmth to the body, for many hundred of years clothing has been used to adorn, to beautify, to exaggerate or otherwise to modify the natural body beautiful. At the same time people—especially women—have carried this to an extreme that is actually unhealthy. Nudist cults still have much going in their favor.

Principal among these atrocities is the girdle. Although in twenty-five years of medical practice I have never seen a woman who would admit to wearing a tight girdle ("I only wear a loose girdle to support my hose"), I have yet to see one where the reddened indentures of the elastic were not obvious on physical examination.

Until recently the wealthy and royal Chinese felt that binding the feet of female infants would give them the beauty symbol of tiny feet. Many such victims could not even walk because of their deformity. As a medical student I recall my anthropology professor bringing to class an armful of human skulls collected from over the world. One was flat on top, produced by binding a board atop the infant's head under the chin so that as the baby grew its skull was quite flat on top—a sign of beauty to that particular tribe. Another skull was quite tall, from the infant's head being bound with a tight band around the forehead, which permitted the growing skull to extend only upward. These were truly bizarre distortions of the human form which to American women would seem ridiculous and absurd, even barbaric—but to those people the American corset or girdle, I daresay, would seem equally ridiculous.

A girdle distorts the female form into a barrel shape without its usual sensuously appealing, graceful contours. For those women who sometimes sneak a peak at *Playboy* and *Penthouse*, the increased number of photographs depicting the derriere is obvious. Few men will deny the erotic "turn-on" of the female buttocks. Even the homosexual woman is excited by such pictures, even more so by the living form. By pressing the buttocks together and bridging the gap between them, a nondescript shape occurs, inhibited in moving grace and having the tactile sensation of a well-inflated basketball. Both below and above this abominable garment occur unsightly bulges which after a long period of time become permanent parts of the figure. The chronic girdle-oholic dismisses any such relationship by calling this "cellulite," a condition unrecognized by the medical fraternity. A most popular, affectionate expression, more so in Italy than in America, is fanny patting in greeting, dancing, and kissing. If used as a premeditated "turn off" or as a modernized version of the chastity belt, the girdle is just right for you!

In addition to its physical abhorrence, both from a visual and tactile standpoint, the girdle constricts the lower abdomen, partially obstructing the return flow of blood from the legs. The venous pressure in the veins of the legs is thereby increased, a condition conducive to unsightly varicose veins. Hemorrhoids, which are merely varicose veins of the rectum and anus, are also more likely to occur. The increased intra-abdominal pressure produced by the girdle tends to expand itself by pushing against all possible areas of least resistance, and in the female this is the pelvic floor. Especially in those women who have borne children, prolapse of the uterus (falling or droppage of the womb) is aided and abetted by the continued onslaught of the unyielding girdle. Hernia of the bladder (cystocele) and rectum (rectocele) into the vagina is usual with uterine prolapse or can occur separately. Once again the increased intra-abdominal pressure conduces to or worsens these conditions. The cystocele may be accompanied by stress incontinence of urine (loss of urinary control when coughing, laughing, running, walking up steps, etc.) and difficulty in voiding. A stagnant pool of urine remains in the herniated bladder which is very prone to infection (cystitis). Rectoceles tend to augment the constipation that most women seem to acquire—I say acquire, because very few people are born with this affliction but by their living habits establish a constipation custom. With large rectoceles it is frequently necessary for the woman to push up on the posterior vaginal wall in order to move her bowels.

In the Gay Nineties the hourglass figure was very much in vogue. The popular stage personality Lillian Russell was one of its greatest champions. Regrettably, she eventually died of a condition called visceroptosis, a falling and constrictive impairment of the function of her visceral organs sufficient to cause death. Although modern garments are not quite so constricting, the same hazards are present, only to a lesser degree.

If you're wearing a girdle because you're too fat, forget it. Your problem is overeating, and a constricting garment is neither healthy nor deceiving. If you really cared how you look, you would not have gotten so fat in the first place. The only person you're fooling is yourself, and you are really the one who needs to face reality. Frankly, my dear, either you don't give a damn or you're so selfish that you want to have your cake and eat it, too!

Everyone knows about the muscular weakness that occurs from chronic illness and disease. If we make the muscles of the abdominal wall rest—and that is exactly what the girdle does—disuse atrophy and weakness occur. The normal function of the anterior abdominal musculature is to hold the abdomen in shape; when denied this use, muscular weakness naturally occurs. It is not uncommon to see women who when dressed (including girdle) have a reasonably flat belly, but when naked have a paunch like a kangaroo with twins. Unfortunately, those who see her in this state of undress are the ones she desires to turn on most—what a disappointment! It reminds me of a story a friend told me about persevering for several months to line up a seemingly very attractive woman he had met. Finally she agreed to go to bed with him. In the process of undressing for the anticipated activity she removed her false eyelashes, her padded brassiere, her false teeth, and her girdle. My friend's state of erect anticipation was superseded by a wave of nausea which, needless to say, rendered him impotent.

For some illogical reason most women after childbirth feel they must immediately don a girdle to conceal their flabby, protruding abdomens. The relaxation is due to the sudden deflation of an overstretched abdominal wall after delivery. With proper exercises, or even just letting the muscles do the work for which they are intended, the tone of the abdominal wall will return in a few weeks. Putting these muscles to rest with a girdle is the best possible way to assure their permanent flaccidity.

Another thought I would like to interject while speaking of childbirth is that there is no known way to prevent stretch marks. Actually they are caused by the stretching of the skin, and layers of the skin separate to produce this condition. There are many salves sold which imply, though not specify, that they can prevent this occurrence. They do not. However, massaging of the skin does stimulate the circulation and can help its elasticity. Baby oil is as good as anything else for this purpose.

Unfortunately, designers and manufacturers of female undergarments are not health conscious or hygienically oriented. Only a fiend could have invented the panty-girdle and panty-hose. No other contribution to human existence could possibly have brought forth the epidemic of female unhygiene caused by these abominations. As a diminutive replica of the girdle, the panty-girdle has the same disadvantages. It has been a causative factor in many gynecologic disorders such as vulvitis (irritation of the vulva), urethritis (inflammation of the tube from the bladder to the outside), and cystitis (infection of the bladder). It is also conducive to varicose veins and swelling of the legs.

In the esoteric circle of gynecologists the term "panty-hose vulvitis" is commonly used. The vulval area, as many other areas of the body, needs fresh air and sunshine in order to flourish. When one wears nylon panties covered by panty-hose, and on top of this a nylon panty-girdle, the lack of air, the stagnation of secretions, and the bacterial fermentation are so conducive to infection that I often wonder how so many women actually escape disease in this area. To further abet this bacterial barrage, some women even sleep in nylon panties to further assure that no air will touch this area! The meager effort by the manufacturer to put a cotton crotch in the nylon garment is a sham, for the nylon on the outside is still present, and, if anything, the circulation of the all-healthful, plain old air is even further restricted. Unquestionably, the most sensible panties for women are those of pure cotton (not the wash-and-wear kind, for the chemicals in these also prevent aeration) and even these should be avoided at night. Perhaps these interjections will help reveal why nudists (or frequent streakers) rarely have vulvitis. There is an age-old medical school saying, "You can't act lovely with pruritus vulvae." It is generally considered unladylike to be constantly scratching this area—your mannerisms may be misinterpreted as masturbation or a pseudostate of nonexistent horniness.

Notice that the purveyors of photographs of sexy women rarely show the nude figure but rather one clad in thigh-high hose and a garter belt. Not only is such an outfit more sensually appealing, but it is actually healthier. (Isn't it indeed pragmatic that sensible and sensuous go together!)

Although the footwear of the younger set is much more anatomically reasonable than that of a decade or more ago, it is still common to see women with corns, bunions, blisters, distortions of the toes, and other foot problems caused by pointed-toed shoes, which have no resemblance to the shape of the human foot. The high- or spike-heeled shoes tend to angulate the pelvic bone in such a manner as to alter appreciably the feminine figure and also impair its natural movement. The constant wearing of high-heeled shoes causes backache and strain to the point that sometimes women are unable to even walk barefooted. All this is rather paradoxical when one considers that the most common fetishes among men are shoes, boots, and feet! Properly fitting shoes that don't bind or otherwise distort or deform the feet will best assure the preservation of this frequently appreciated, erogenous area. Always buy shoes late in the afternoon when any swelling of the feet occurring during the day has already had time to manifest itself. Whether you realize it or not, whenever you're swimming or otherwise barefooted, your feet are under careful scrutiny, so keep them clean, the nails properly trimmed and their shape intact. Pretty feet are an asset. Don't abuse them —keep them kissable!

CHAPTER 2

Bras and Breasts

I HAVE some good news and some bad news. The annihilation of bras by the women's liberation movement is both good and bad. There is no question that the artificial support of the budding breast impairs the organic function of the supporting connective tissues of the breasts (Cooper's ligaments). Although the breast has no muscular support, and no known exercises will enlarge or shape it, the connective tissue supports will lose tone when completely resting in the horrendous hammock of the bra. Most assuredly the most oppressive use of this instrument is by the overly protective mother who insists that her ten- to twelve-year-old daughter wear a brassiere. The only possible result of such admonition is to make the child self-conscious about her breast development—either large or small—and to impose upon her an undeserved guilt complex about this area of her body.

I am not opposed to bras, nor do I favor them. Large or pendulous breasts obviously need support. The very weight of the breast itself can strain its ligamentous supports. The nursing mother needs support for the lactating breast. Perhaps there is still no better way to decide one's need for this garment than the "pencil test." Place a pencil horizontally under your breast. Stand up. If the pencil falls, you don't need a bra.

Disadvantages of the bra include restriction of the circulation and impairment of the natural development of the nipple and the breast configuration. The natural movement of the breast, which is sensuously stimulating to men and to the woman as well, is restricted; and particularly in the obese person with pendulous breasts, undue perspiration with its accompanying odor can result. Long-term use of this garment can alter the sensitivity of the breast, sometimes to the point of loss of feeling.

It is of interest that among the tribes where bras are unknown and breasts are bared, sagginess or droppage so common in the United States is less frequent, except in those women who have undergone repeated pregnancy and lactation without support.

Most women are especially self-conscious about their breasts—as men are about their penises. Unfortunately, many are dissatisfied with either the size, shape, configuration or nipple orientation. An inferiority complex or even anxiety neurosis can sometimes be based on woman's preoccupation with her breasts. Also it is not uncommon to encounter women who have one breast larger than the other, another cause of considerable concern.

Fortunately, now with the miracles of modern surgery, breast augmentation and diminution can be performed very safely and effectively. With proper surgical techniques, large, pendulous breasts can be altered to almost any size and configuration. Also by the use of silicone implants, those women unhappily endowed can be revitalized to the size they desire. By silicone implants I mean the plastic-encased silicone bags. Injections of silicone into the breast can be very dangerous from the standpoint of infection, necrosis, and even cancer.

Even before the turn of the century surgical attempts at breast augmentation were undertaken with prostheses of sponges, ivory, wood and other materials. Later injections of paraffin and other waxes were used to enlarge the female breast; however, severe complications from necrosis or tumor formation such as the well-known "paraffinoma" occurred. In the last several decades much progress has been made in breast augmentation operations. The development of polyester plastics, which produce little or no tissue reaction, has paved the way to a reasonably safe, simple, and very effective method of accomplishing the desired result—namely a permanently beautiful and graceful breast with little or no loss of its sexual sensitivity and lactational function.

At the present time the most popular method of breast augmentation surgery is to implant a plastic pouch which is then inflated, or one which is already inflated, with a silicone gel. These operations leave only small scars, usually below the fold under the breast, which are hardly visible. Although yet far from perfect, the silicone pouch is the safest, most effective method of breast enlargement.

Before considering a silicone implant, a woman should be aware of some medical aspects. To be sure, some men are aroused by large breasts, but some are not. If this is a big source of dissension between you and your husband, then consider the advantages of the operation. On the other hand, many men are not breast freaks and breast size is not too important to them. If your man is one of these, forget it! Artificial breasts do not always look like breasts and they don't always feel like breasts, but improvements in surgical techniques and prosthesis design are rapidly overcoming these drawbacks.

The one thing that most women, and men, too, for that matter, don't realize is that the number of sensory nerve endings in the breast is the same, regardless of its size. As a matter of fact, women with small breasts are usually more sensitive in this area than those with large breasts. In the operation for silicone implantation, there is some risk of severing the breast's sensory nerves, but not usually. On the other hand, many women derive a tremendous psychological lift from this procedure, which overcomes many of its disadvantages. Most women who have had either breast augmentation or reduction operations report an increased interest in and responsiveness to sexual activity. Neither silicone implants nor breast reduction operations necessarily interfere with the basic breast function of lactation and breast feeding, a source of considerable maternal satisfaction as well as a vicarious sexual stimulation to most women.

The mammaplastic operations done for large and pendulous breasts are quite satisfactory. Usually these require a reimplantation of the nipple and removal of the excess tissue below this point through an incision beneath the breasts. The scar is not readily visible. I once saw a famous movie star's wife who had had such an operation, and she said that her husband never knew it!

If you're contemplating either operation, think clearly before you rush into it. Don't concentrate your whole evaluation of your self-esteem on the size of your breasts. After all this is a relatively small part of your body. If you do decide to have breast augmentation or reduction surgery, have a competent plastic surgeon do the procedure. Ask your family doctor or specialist to recommend a qualified surgeon. You can also contact the county medical association, a nearby teaching hospital, or the *Directory of Medical Specialists*, which is available in most public libraries.

It would be impossible to estimate the untold millions of dollars American women spend each year for "quack" products for breast enlargement. Such methods as hormone creams (which may contain only traces of female hormones), aphrodisiac diets, suction cups, and exercises are considered medically ineffective and sometimes dangerous. (For men who are reading this book, I might also add that there is no known way to enlarge the penis and all advertisements of ways and means of accomplishing the same are completely phony!) The exercises for breast enlargement merely enlarge the pectoral muscles (the muscles underneath the breast), but not the size of the breast. The larger suction pumps, which are sold for breast enlargement, produce trauma, congestion with blood and thus temporary swelling, but no long-term benefit is possible.

It is perhaps paradoxical that large doses of estrogen (female hormone) in males produce breast enlargement, but the same is not usually true for women. Sometimes however, one does encounter women who will experience breast enlargement from estrogen as occasionally occurs with birth control pills. The effect here is similar to pregnancy, which sometimes enlarges breasts and sometimes not. Recently there have been claims by some women that ingestion of semen during fellation increases the size of their breasts. The prostaglandin (a form of hormone) content of semen could possibly produce this effect in those individuals whose breasts are hormonally responsive. There are medical reports that demonstrate enlargement of the male breast from marijuana, but unfortunately the same effect does not occur in women.

One question with which I am constantly confronted is the effect of pregnancy, lactation, and nursing on the size and tone of the breasts and what influence these functions may have on the development of cancer of the breast. In a word, the answer should be none and none. More specifically, it is not unusual to see some atrophy (shrinkage) of the breast after pregnancy whether or not the baby is breast-fed. However, in a few months after normal menstruation and hormone balance resume, I do not find, in general, any difference in the breasts of women who have or have not nursed their babies. Of course, suitable support should be used during pregnancy and lactation, so that the supportive, connective tissues of the breast do not become overstretched and lax. It is certainly not possible for even the most astute gynecologist to examine a woman several years after childbirth and tell whether or not she nursed a child! Furthermore, there is no evidence that pregnancy and lactation increase the incidence of cancer of the breast; some studies even show the contrary to be true.

Another breast problem that confronts many women is inverted nipples. Paradoxically their concern frequently leads to an inhibitory shyness about their nipples to the point that they actually avoid the very activities which could help overcome this condition, namely sucking, pinching, or other tactile stimulation which cause the nipple to erect. Almost always the erect nipple protrudes; therefore, any activity that stimulates this effect is helpful and should be carried out several times a day. In addition to the above, cold water applied to the nipple areas will usually cause them to erect. For women with this problem the usual bra is not indicated. Either a French-type nude bra that goes around the breast with the nipple portion exposed, or a bra with holes cut in it to expose the nipple, would be much better. This permits constant stimulation of the nipple by the outer clothing. The prolonged or unduly frequent use of a breast pump, such as is used by nursing mothers, can occasionally cause injury to the breast. Don't feel you're a freak because of your inverted problem. As with many other psychological hang-ups the best way to solve your problem is to let it all hang out, and in no instance can I think this adage is more appropriate than with inverted nipples. The very hang-out may solve your hang-up and its basic cause as well. Don't play like the ostrich that avoids all worldly problems by sticking its head in the sand. The only way to solve a problem is to bring it out into the open, and in the case of the breast nipples, to bare it.

CHAPTER 3

The Vapor Trail

IF it's a spray, it's hell to pay—not the obliteration of the ozone layer above the earth which protects us from the barrage of deadly ultraviolet radiation, but the damage—both physical and psychological—that occurs from their use. Since the sinister pseudo-ingenious development of the spray can, everything imaginable has been merchandised in this medium. Aside from the paints, glues, oven cleaners, and nonstick pan preparations, the products offered for feminine alterations are both hygienically inappropriate and aesthetically objectionable. The worst of these is the so-called "feminine hygiene spray." I was delighted to read recently that these products soon must have a warning label and the words "hygiene" or "hygienic" deleted from the labels and advertisements. The Food and Drug Administration deserves an "A" for this effort; actually these products have no medicinal value whatsoever.

Utterly abominable in their olfactory permeations, these sprays can and do cause frequent vulval irritations. First, the most aphrodisiac odor to the human male is the aroma of the female vagina. Everyone knows the way a male dog first smells and licks the female before the anticipated sexual encounter. This same olfactory savoring is true of most animals, and the human is no different. Ads in underground newspapers frequently have worn panties for sale, and some women sell as many as a hundred pairs a week merely because the fragrant, sensuous aroma of the female vagina is a definite "turn on" for most males. The male purchaser of this item inhales the aromatic essence and uses it for stimulation and fantasy during masturbation. So it is capriciously naïve for a woman to replace an olfactory attribute which has everything going for it, with the odor of lemon-lime, strawberry, or lilac. I have never known any of these fragrances to be sensually stimulating to men. If your lover is a strawberry freak, why tantalize him with the distaste and pseudo-smell of artificial strawberry flavoring? Put some fresh strawberries in your vagina so he can relish the real thing!

Whereas most users of these atomized abominations think they're turning men on, actually they're doing exactly the opposite. But worst of all is the vulval irritation caused by the chemicals in the spray and the aerosol propellant. Hygiene sprays had hardly hit the market when I began to see patients with vulval irritations from them. Actually, a high percentage of women who use sprays have *irritation from them.*

Absorption of the propellant from the vagina and the inhalation of its fumes can cause damage to the heart and lungs. A recent case was reported in which a young girl had inhaled the vapor and died. Whether or not this was done as an intentional suicide or accidentally we'll never know, but at least it points out the extent of the hazards of the spray.

It is interesting to observe that the primary users of the sprays are young girls, ages sixteen to twenty, who think they are really "with it." Once again the hucksters have triumphed over gullible, unlearned innocence.

The next line of offense in the waging of chemical warfare against the natural beauty of the feminine form is the hair spray. This dilute glue or lacquer fixes the hair in any undesirable configuration imaginable and gives the hair a texture about the same as 00 steel wool.

Some years ago I saw a patient who complained of shortness of breath and difficult breathing. She was a beautician, and in the course of each day she inhaled untold amounts of hair spray. As it fixes the hair, it also fixes the lungs, and despite innumerable warnings as to the dangers of such products, women still use them in abundance. I advised this beautician to discontinue this affront to her lungs or suffer permanent pulmonary damage, but of course she refused. Surely the inhalation of such vapors can only be damaging over the years, probably far worse than the inhalation of tobacco smoke.

One of my patients was a pregnant lady complaining of nausea and vomiting. On further questioning I learned that this was not the usual morning sickness, but rather it occurred only when she used hair spray. She was a large woman with her hair teased into a gross bouffant, and she really looked like a refugee from a cartoon carnival. When I suggested an instant, obvious solution to her problem, she replied, "But what could I do with my hair?" Frankly, if she had gone and soaked her head, it could not have looked any worse.

It has always been puzzling to me to try to analyze the motivation of women to compliment each other on their hairdos. No doubt jealousy, sarcasm, envy, and pity enter into the possibilities or probabilities, but most of all I think it is the age-old story that misery loves company, and seeing others submit to this form of torture further justifies—even abets—their own rationale for this miserable abuse.

CHAPTER 4

Spring Cleaning

SEVERAL years ago I was having a party of about twelve couples at my river cabin one wintry evening. The temperature was twenty degrees. One of the ladies arrived reeking to the high heavens with the most pungent, acrid perfume I had ever smelled —she really must have bathed in it. The room was so asphyxiating that all the men stayed out on the porch in freezing weather rather than endure the olfactory offense. I'm sure this woman thought she was really "uptown" with her fancy perfume and her mink stole, but even a skunk couldn't have caused more revulsion. No doubt some pinheaded clerk in a department store had convinced her that it was the latest thing.

Perfumes, like garlic, must be used sparingly and with appropriate judiciousness in order to be appreciated. Unfortunately there are now products for men which are equally as stifling. Like one who has chronic B.O., the excessive user of perfumes becomes immune to the odor and its offensiveness to others. For some reason it is considered impolite and an invasion of privacy to tell a person that she has B.O., and even more so to tell one that her perfume stinks.

The most common offenders in the aroma arena are teeny-boppers and middle-aged women, the former because of their gullibility for advertisements, hucksterism, and salesmanship, such as for a new kind of crunchy, fruity, breakfast cereal, and the latter because their olfactory organs have been numbed by many years' exposure. As the deafening din of acid rock has been proven to be detrimental to the hearing, constant exposure to highly aromatic essences tends to deaden the delicate appreciation of subtle, delectable—even tantalizing natural odors that should appeal to the erotic sensations of interpersonal relationships.

I keep room deodorants in my office, for occasionally they are desirable. Only once in twenty-five years have I had to use one because of a patient's B.O., but frequently they are necessary to subdue the permeating stench of cheap, overpowering perfumes.

Except for the rarely encountered condition of hyperhidrosis (excessive sweating), most body odor can be controlled with simple bathing, particularly after strenuous exercise or work. Deodorant soaps are neither helpful nor advisable for this. Many of them are not soaps at all, but detergents which cause excessive dryness and irritation to the skin, while others contain potent and harsh chemicals which are only weakly bacteriocidal and probably kill mostly the harmless bacteria that normally cover the skin, rather than many forms of disease-causing germs that may be present.

The currently available products for body deodorization have no effect against the gram-negative colon bacillus that normally covers the vulva, nor do they have an effect against fungus. Actually, the use of such agents in this area may make the user more susceptible to fungus infections! Most skin is very tough and can endure much insult, but the delicate mucous membranes of the vulva are more sensitive and usually will be the first area to react against the use of deodorant soaps. For example, one can apply vinegar to the hand, arm, and body with very little irritation, but just try putting vinegar on the vulva—you'll think it's on fire!

Deodorant soaps had been on the market hardly a month when I began to see vulval irritation caused by them. It has been my custom to ask every woman I see what kind of soap she uses, and this inquiry has revealed a causal relationship to innumerable cases of irritative vulvitis. Another disadvantage to deodorant soaps is the occasional problem of photosensitivity, a condition that can make one more susceptible to severe sunburn. Even severe blistering and swelling can occur with minimal exposure to sunlight in the habitual user of these soaps, and suntan lotions do not protect against this hazard.

For those who are convinced that they suffer from B.O., a mild soap and an antiperspirant—perhaps even one with an antiseptic—should work better than "deodorant soaps."

Dermatologists contend that most people bathe too frequently and that water is bad for the skin. I have even read reports in the medical journals by dermatologists recommending that people bathe no oftener than every two weeks. This may be too infrequent for most of us, but on the other hand, many people—especially women—have obsessive compulsions to bathe two, three, or more times a day when they have been under no exertion to cause sweating and consequent B.O. This is ridiculous and harmful to the health and texture of the skin. People should bathe when they need to, either because they're dirty or because of considerable perspiration produced by exertion.

In reality, fresh perspiration has a very subtle odor, actually an aphrodisiac to most people. It has been said that the great Casanova, master of amorous conquests, would carry his handkerchief in his armpit and then offer it to a lady to wipe her face. To some extent his seductive success was attributed to that ruse.

Most people will admit that the fragrance of fresh perspiration such as occurs during intercourse is a definite "turn on." To be sure, the subtle, natural odor of some bodies do not appeal to the sensuous inhalations of another, but also the shape of the face, or for that matter the whole body itself, might be unattractive. Unfortunately, the human has the poorest sense of smell of any mammal, and many times sensory perception of odors is at a subconscious level, such that incompatibility of human body aromas can rarely be defined.

It is the fermentation of perspiration that causes the odor, and this takes several hours. To acquire a really fulminating case of B.O. takes several days but, in any event, the cure is not with deodorant soaps or perfumes. Simple washing with a mild soap is all that is necessary. Many soaps are so overly perfumed as to be aromatically objectionable. Ads which state that they make one smell clean are as ridiculous as trying to describe the aroma of fresh air. What does "clean" smell like? Normally people smell good as good people should, but an artificial aroma is really just another form of hypocrisy.

From a more realistic viewpoint, many so-called deodorant soaps are not really soaps at all, but detergents which by their very detergent action tend to remove the natural oils from the body skin. (If you will check the labels carefully, some say "Beauty Deodorant Bar.") If you suffer from dry skin, first of all avoid excessive bathing, but most of all avoid deodorant soaps and detergents. And of the latter, the worst offender is the "bubble bath." They are detergents which make pretty bubbles, but they aggravate your skin problem.

Because of persistent persecution by the various media, many women are now convinced that they are the most odorous animals on the earth. Thus the boulevard is paved for the mass merchandising of all sorts of deodorant preparations—breath deodorants, armpit deodorants, overall body deodorants, vaginal deodorants, foot deodorants, etc., ad nauseam. On of the most frequent hang-ups I see in my office is woman complaining of abnormal and offensive odors—even to the point of paranoid obsession with this idea. And of course the most frequent source of the odor is the vagina. Although the normal, healthy vagina does not produce an unpleasant odor, I find it extremely difficult to convince patients that their fears are unfounded. Frequently after removing the vaginal speculum from these women, I place it under their noses so that they can confirm for themselves that there is no objectionable odor. Actually, any unpleasant odor from the normal female perineum is produced *outside* the vagina by the fermentation of perspiration and other secretions by the bacterial flora of the vulva, usually the colon bacillus.

Bacteria are like cowboys—there are good guys and bad guys. Many unknowledgeable people feel that all bacteria are harmful and fail to understand the benevolent acts of the "good guys." About 60 percent of our digestion is due to the fermentative action of bacteria. The balance of microorganisms in our environment is the main reason we are not already extinct from the infestation of numerous deadly germs. For some years it was the usual practice of pediatricians to order daily baths of babies with hexachlorophene soaps (such as Phisohex) in order to try to avoid the pathogenic organism, *Staphylococcus aureus*. Subsequent experience revealed permanent brain damage in so many babies from hexachlorophene that now the F.D.A. has removed it from the over-the-counter market. Unfortunately, rendering the babies' (or anyone's, for that matter) skin free of bacteria is sort of like plowing under—or otherwise destroying—a good strand of grass. What can be expected is an overgrowth of weeds, or, in more microscopic terms, a takeover by disease germs. The skin, intestinal tract, and particularly the vagina are covered with harmless—even helpful—bacteria and to eradicate them by any means opens the door to the invasion of the more harmful bacteria or fungi that cause disease. It is not realistically possible or even hygienically advantageous to try to approach a bacteria-free environment. We must think of some microorganisms as pets, friends, or colleagues. To destroy them is to destroy ourselves.

DEODORIZING ANALYSING

Who would want to deodorize a rose, the fine bouquet of a well-aged wine, or a woman? Nevertheless, the covetous market for deodorants, antiperspirants, and masking perfumes appeals to the vast majority of our populace, especially women.

Antiperspirants inhibit perspiration, a normal and healthy bodily function. By eliminating perspiration it is presumed that B.O. can thereby be controlled. However, it is not the volume of the sweat that causes the odor, but the duration of its existence and the extent of its bacterial fermentation.

The other approach to altering the normal aroma of the body is the use of deodorants which attempt to eliminate the odor of perspiration, rather than stop its secretion by killing the bacteria which ferment it. Needless to say, neither of these approaches can surpass the need for cleanliness. A little soap and water can readily eliminate the undesirable emanations and at the same time remove any dirt or grime that may be present and permit the true individual essence to prevail.

Antiperspirants are usually made up of aluminum compounds like chlorides and chlorhydroxides. To many people these are irritating and can cause severe skin rashes. Deodorants contain antibacterial agents in the form of powder, pastes, creams, roll-ons, and aerosol sprays. There is no advantage to the spray can as a means of applying deodorants. If you do insist on using them, the prolonged inhalation of these vapors can cause lung disease.

Over the years I have seen many cases of women who have shaved their armpits and then applied deodorant pastes or creams. These actually plug up the skin pores, causing infection of the glands under the arms so painful that these women have to walk with their arms outstretched. Sometimes these infections abscess, and incision and drainage with antibiotic therapy is necessary.

Don't lose your individual odor—it's part of your character.

HAIR CARE

Contrary to popular belief, dandruff is not a disease, an infection, or a curable condition. It is merely a shedding of the scalp skin cells, the same as shedding of dead skin cells all over the body that occurs all the time in everyone. Some people are afflicted with this problem more than others, but everyone has it to a greater or lesser extent. So-called dandruff-removing shampoos are no better than ordinary shampoos—or even soap—for removing the cellular debris. Actually, some detergent shampoos, by causing excessive dehydration and drying of the scalp, may even increase the shedding—to wit, dandruff!

Another commercialized consideration worthy of condemnation is the so-called protein additive in shampoos. As hair above the skin surface is really *dead*, nothing applied to it will revitalize or otherwise alter it any more than trying to bring a dead person back to life.

May I also add that lemon juice, eggs, and beer, other than adding their particular aroma, have no value in hair care.

Since people vary tremendously in the oiliness of their skin and hair, the frequency of hair washing is an individual problem. If the hair is very oily, it needs washing frequently. On the other hand, people with dry skin and dandruff need to wash it as rarely as possible. Only when the accumulation of dandruff becomes objectionable should the hair be shampooed, for too frequent washings will surely cause worsening of the dandruff deluge.

In the field of cosmetic commercialism unquestionably 99 44/100 percent of it is 100 percent bunkum. Eyebrow extenders, fingernail hardeners, natural beauty aids, skin conditioners, and facial improvers probably cause more harm than good by causing frequent chemical and allergic reactions, but worst of all, they fail to give the allure that the ads insure.

DISHPAN HANDS

Properly called detergent dermatitis, this is all too commonly an affliction of women. Househusbands rarely suffer from this problem simply because they practically never do the dishes. The dry, reddened, blistered, and fissured appearance of the skin is characteristic of this condition. Despite the commercial commendation of numerous products, there are none that won't cause this trouble. Yet, strangely enough, many women fail to recognize the causal relationship. It is a frequent retort, when I render this diagnosis, to hear, "But doctor, it can't be that because I only use 'Cueball' liquid, which is good for the hands." It is true that some of these products do soften the skin—so much so that it peels, cracks—and later becomes dry and rough and loses the feel that men—or even women, love to touch. This reaction occurs particularly under rings, where inadequate rinsing fails to remove all traces of the chemical irritant. All too frequently this is presumed to be an allergy to the metal in the ring itself. The appearance, the texture, and softness of hands are some of woman's greatest attributes and should be preserved at all costs. A dishwashing machine is really cheap when compared to the cost of prolonged dermatologic treatment of a self-induced disease. If your husband is too tight, impecunious, or otherwise refuses to buy you a machine, then insist that he do the dishes; and if this fails, remedy the situation by wearing rubber gloves. The problem with this, however, is that usually the dishwater and detergent seep in over the rubber gloves; therefore, the same hazard is present.

The application of various hand lotions cannot cure or overcome the persistent persecution imposed by dishwashing detergents. Although few of the modern generation realize it, dishes can be washed with mild soap and water—and just as effectively, if you're doing them by hand! This could merit you a favorable factor in avoiding the dilemma of "dishpan hands."

BAD BREATH

Probably there is no more common obsession promulgated upon our society than the generalized fear of having bad breath (halitosis). The American public spends several hundred millions of dollars per year for nostrums to correct this, usually imaginary, condition. For the most part, all of this "junk" is worthless for any more than very temporary alterations of breath odors. Products containing chlorophyll or antiseptics have no lasting benefit. The human mouth contains a tremendous variety of bacteria, and no mouthwash or lozenge will sterilize this area. Oral surgeons well know the futility of trying to render the mouth bacteria-free, for when they perform operations inside the mouth no effort is made to sterilize the field. The mouth is amazingly immune to infection, particularly by its own bacteria.

It is true that some bad breath occurs from fermentation of food particles between the teeth and in the mouth, but the solution is to clean the teeth with brush, dental floss or water pick, and not to try to kill the bacteria. Gargling with salt or plain water is as effective as any mouthwash in cleansing the mouth and soothing the throat. Furthermore, the commercially available products have no value whatsoever in preventing or curing colds or sore throats.

Physical causes of halitosis include such conditions as tooth decay, pyorrhea, tonsillitis and other throat infections, and diseases of the lung and intestinal tract. These require proper diagnosis and treatment by your physician or dentist. A mouthwash is not the answer.

Smoking, drinking, and eating aromatic foods such as garlic or onions may impart an objectionable odor to your breath. Thus if you anticipate an amorous adventure, it would be best to avoid these offenders unless your partner also indulges.

Why it is so many people (especially women) dislike their bodies, the color of their hair, the shape of their faces, the length and shape of their legs, their breasts, their eyes, their thighs, their toes and nose, and for that matter, *themwholeselves* is hard to fathom. Unquestionably, however, a big, big factor in the creation of inferiority feelings is the commercial confrontation experienced every time one opens a periodical, turns on TV, or listens to the radio. True, the sexy shape, the sensuous voice, and the shapely form of the models hustling various products are indeed appealing, but what they don't say is that if you use their products, you will *not* look the same, sound the same, or have the same degree of sex appeal. I once knew a woman who ate the same diet that Lily Pons did, thinking that it would make her sing like Lily Pons. She couldn't and she never will. Using striped paint will not make you a zebra, nor spotted paint a leopard.

Beauty in all living things has four dimensions—color, shape, texture, and aroma. If any, or particularly all, of these dimensions is false, one becomes as an artificial, imitation, fake reproduction of a Rembrandt—worthless. Undoubtedly there are some men who are impressed by artificial, flamboyant hair styles and indelicately painted faces, but there are also men who can appreciate zircons as if they were diamonds, red glass as rubies, and brass as gold.

If people could just be themselves, not filled with petty jealousies and unjust inferiority feelings, they would be infinitely better off. Regardless of your greatest attributes, whether they be in beauty, knowledge, artistic ability, or otherwise, unless you are prodigious, there is always someone in the world who can surpass you. It is not possible for everyone to stand on the top rung of the ladder. Happiness is being yourself, doing your own thing, not pretending to be something or someone you're not, and most of all, loving living as it is. Probably you're better looking than you think, smarter than you think, and sexier than you think!

CHAPTER 5

The Vagina and Its Adversaries

NORMALLY the adult vagina is inhabited by *Lactobacillus acidophilus*, the very same bacteria found in every glass of milk we drink. The souring of milk is only a process of fermentation by these bacteria. In the vagina similar bacteria ferment the glycogen in the vaginal mucous membranes, producing lactic acid. This acid environment of the vagina makes it very resistant to disease-causing germs.

As early as 1895 Kronig, a German gynecologist, experimented with female prison volunteers as to the susceptibility of the vagina to disease-causing germs. He found the normal, healthy vagina to be very resistant to disease, even gonorrhea. However, in another group of volunteers whom Kronig had take daily douches and then put the same germs in the vagina, the disease rate was very high. Yet today, eighty years later, women still use douches for so-called "cleanliness." The only action of the douche is to wash out the friendly bacteria and the lactic acid and hence, susceptibility to infection is greatly increased. In addition to the increased susceptibility to infection, the douche causes excessive dryness of the vagina by washing out its normal secretions which are so important in providing proper lubrication for intercourse.

I once saw a patient in her late forties who complained of such severe dyspareunia (painful intercourse) because of dryness that she had been unable to have intercourse for one and a half years. She had consulted her family physician, who logically reasoned that if she had excessive dryness, she should wet it; so he prescribed two douches daily. After this failed to work, he advised three douches daily. Needless to say, this didn't work either. After this I was consulted. I advised the patient to take no more douches and return in two weeks. When she returned, she stated that she was perfectly well and was then enjoying normal sexual relations without discomfort.

Advertisements of douche preparations in most women's magazines and on TV would give the impression that the normal vagina stinks. This is not true. The secretions of the normal vagina and vulva have a very subtle, unobjectionable aroma which has the most aphrodisiac effect on men of any odor, natural or artificial, in the world. To replace this with the scent of mint, eucalyptus, or perfume is to destroy one of the most vital female attributes. Please note that the above comments apply to the normal, healthy vagina; certain vaginal infections, especially trichomonas vaginitis, can produce an extremely fetid, foul, acrid, and nauseating odor. There is no douche that will either prevent or cure vaginal infections. In twenty-five years of practicing gynecology, I have never found douches even helpful in the treatment of any vaginal infection; and women who regularly take douches invariably have more vaginal infections than those who do not. As a matter of fact, I have cured many cases of vaginal discharge merely by having the patient stop douching. It is not uncommon to see women actually irritated by many douche preparations.

Many women have the feeling that douching after intercourse is an absolute *must* for feminine hygiene. I don't know what they imagine the vagina is like inside after intercourse, but they obviously think its pretty terrible. In the management of cases of infertility, one of the commonly used tests has the woman come to the office as soon as possible after intercourse without douching; a specimen is made from the vagina to evaluate the relative number and motility of the sperm. When performing these tests, you would be surprised how difficult it is to get one drop of material to put on a slide for microscopic examination! After intercourse the vagina neither smells bad nor teems with seminal ebullience.

Many years ago I was on emergency duty when a young woman who had been raped by six men was brought in by the police. The girl was distraught and incoherent. However, on examination I was impressed with the healthy, normal appearance of the vagina. Thus one could conclude that repeated intercourse is not harmful to the vagina, but is actually healthy! This concept is further borne out by gynecologists who have examined many prostitutes and concluded that intercourse per se is not harmful to the vagina or pelvic organs.

The effects of douching on fertility have long been a topic of fervent debate in gynecologic circles. As a contraceptive the douche is particularly ineffective (even if used immediately after intercourse). On the other hand, by destroying the normal vaginal environment, the douche can be a factor in infertility. I have always discouraged the use of the douche for women who want to become pregnant. Others have claimed that acid (vinegar) douches prior to intercourse are conducive to male offspring and alkaline (soda) douches are conducive to female, but as yet there is insufficient data to substantiate this concept.

For douching, the bulb syringe is potentially dangerous, especially during pregnancy. Many cases of air embolism from this instrument have been reported. (Air embolism is a condition caused by air entering the bloodstream—in this situation through the lining of the womb—and going to the heart. The heartbeat then only contracts the air and pumps no blood, so death occurs.) Numerous cases of air embolism during pregnancy have also been reported from blowing into the vagina during oral sexual activity.

With regard to the so-called cleansing or hygienic suppositories, the substitutes for douches, these have the same unbeneficial properties as the douches so adequately covered above. The one exception is that some "hygiene" suppositories are very strong spermatocides (contraceptives), but because some states still outlaw the prescription or sale of contraceptives, they are not advertised as such.

Vaginal tampons for use during menstruation have, since their introduction, been a controversial topic in gynecologic circles. As to my own experience they are without merit except for occasional use for a few hours during athletic events, swimming, etc. Most women who use them regularly experience more pain and more flow during the period and have a brownish discharge following the period. I have often examined women a day or two after the period and found fragments of cotton lint in the vagina which cause a foreign body focus for infection and a foul discharge. The absorbency of the tampon soaks up not only the menstrual blood, but also the vaginal secretions, which causes an excessive dryness of the vagina, an impairment to intercourse for several days following the period. Like any foreign body the tampon with its ideal culture medium—the menstrual blood—makes a perfect environment for infection, and as a matter of fact, this can and does frequently occur. There is no fouler and repulsive odor and discharge that emits from the human vagina than that from a tampon that has been left in for two or more weeks—a condition I see all too often!

By blocking the free flow of menstruation, the tampon causes accumulation of menstrual fluid within the womb, which in turn contracts (cramps) more actively in order to empty itself. This causes an increase in pain, and the womb distended with blood bleeds more into itself, causing an increased flow. The entrapped blood within the womb decomposes into brownish blood by-products and drains for days after the period is over. The entrapped blood once again is conducive to infection, and inflammation of the lining of the womb may occur.

In one six-month period I had three college girls, all virgins who regularly used tampons, consult me concerning persistent bleeding for six to eight weeks. When D and Cs (scraping the lining from the womb) were done, chronic infection of the lining of the womb was found in each case. As tampons were the only things they had had in the vagina, it was only logical to presume a causal relationship.

In the bacteriology laboratory we grow bacteria at a temperature of 98.6 degrees (normal body temperature) on blood agar plates covered to exclude air. When one realizes that these experimental conditions are almost identical to the environment of the menstruating woman with a tampon, it makes one wonder why infections with its use are not even more common.

Although there are differences of opinion, many gynecologists feel that tampons are a factor in the causation of endometriosis, a very serious disease characterized by the growth of the lining tissue of the womb that bleeds with menstruation, outside the confines of the uterine cavity. The cause of this disease has been proved to be retrograde menstruation—bleeding out through the fallopian tubes instead of the vagina. The menstrual fluid contains living cells from the lining of the womb, and these cells can implant themselves and grow on the ovaries, in the pelvis, on the bowel, or wherever they land.

Textbooks of gynecology twenty years ago described endometriosis as a disease mainly of women thirty-five years of age or older, but recently I have seen many cases of women in their twenties, some unmarried with little or no sexual experience, seriously afflicted with this disease. Last year I had a twenty-two-year-old patient with extensive endometriosis involving both ovaries, fallopian tubes, and pelvis requiring complete removal of these organs. For a young woman who had never been pregnant, this was a very traumatic experience. She had used tampons for seven years. Although this was not a proved causation, it at least raised some doubt in the mind of the most critical observer.

In a patient only twenty-four years old, I found not only the above evidences of disease but two areas of intestinal obstruction requiring resection of the bowel as well as removal of the pelvic organs. Once again the history of the use of tampons was of many years' duration.

The causative mechanism of endometriosis by backflow of menstrual fluid through the tubes has been well proven by the rhesus monkey experiments of Dr. Roger Scott, but it took several years for the disease to develop, even when the womb was reversed so that it menstruated directly into the abdominal cavity. The significance of this observation is merely that if you use tampons today and don't have endometriosis next week, don't conclude that there is no harmful potential of this otherwise extolled convenience.

I am well aware of the occasional chafing and irritation of the usual sanitary napkins for menstrual hygiene, but nowadays so many women are on birth control pills and have such a light menstrual flow because of them that for many the minipad is adequate protection.

The other side of the tampon coin is the familiarity of a woman with her genitalia, her awareness of the vagina. The frequent use of tampons tends to minimize the reflexive contraction of the vaginal muscles—the condition called vaginismus. This prior conditioning of the vagina also makes one's first intercourse less painful and pelvic examinations, so necessary in continuing female health, less traumatic, both physically and psychologically. As with many other aspects of living, good judgment rather than an all-or-none approach must be used with tampons.

If you must use tampons, avoid those that are perfumed and contain deodorants. Totally ineffectual in their advertised advantages, they frequently cause allergic and chemical irritations which vitiate any other possible desirability of such trash.

CHAPTER 6

V.D. and Other Bad News

WARNING: Sexual activity may be hazardous to your health! The surgeon general's admonition which appears on every pack of cigarettes that smoking may be hazardous to your health is in fact a warning against a relatively small facet of total human disease. The incidence and seriousness of V.D. (now preferably called Sexually Transmitted Disease [S.T.D.]) is far greater than any consequences of cigarette smoking. Perhaps the government will some day pass laws requiring every woman to wear a label on her mons veneris and every man to have tattooed on his penis—"This can be hazardous to your health!"

Although most all sexual activities among healthy people are generally harmless, notwithstanding the risk of pregnancy, there are a number of diseases which can be and are transmitted by sexual activity.

SYPHILIS

The titan of V.D. is syphilis. The noted physician Sir William Osler once said that he who knows syphilis knows all of medicine, for syphilis is the great masquerader—it can mimic any disease of the human body. Commonly referred to as "syph," "lues," "pox," or "bad blood," syphilis is caused by a spirochetal germ called the *Treponema pallidum.* Although generally contracted through sexual intercourse, syphilis can be caused by noncoital means such as simple kissing or contact with open cuts or abrasions on the skin. Syphilis is considered to be an occupational disease among doctors, nurses, and prostitutes. Although the disease is very contagious in certain stages, such implausible sources as drinking glasses, dishes, toilet seats and swimming pools are hardly acceptable prevarications or explanation.

The primary lesion of syphilis is the chancre, a hard ulcer one-fourth to three-fourths inch in diameter, usually singular and not tender. In the male the most common location of the lesion is the penis, but chancres can and do occur on every part of the human body. The lips, mouth, anus, breasts, even hands and toes are not unusual sites. In the female, however, the primary lesion is frequently in the vagina or on the cervix, and because of the minimal symptoms it produces, usually goes undetected.

The average time after exposure for the chancre to appear is three weeks, but it can be anywhere from ten to ninety days. In this early stage the blood test is negative—it takes about six weeks for the blood test to become positive. The syphilitic nature of the primary lesion, however, can be positively identified by special microscopic examination of scrapings from the ulcer.

Whether treated or not, the chancre will disappear in about four to six weeks, and the patient will seem apparently well until the secondary stage of the disease occurs, anywhere from six weeks to six months. The typical secondary lesion is a generalized red raised skin rash, frequently covering the whole body. Usually there is no itching. Other manifestations of the secondary stage include local areas of baldness (even loss of eyebrows and eyelashes), mucus patches on the mouth or other moist areas, and flat warts (condylomata lata) in the anogenital area.

Once again as with the primary lesion, the secondary signs will disappear in two to six weeks. Then the disease goes into a latent or quiescent stage that can last one to twenty years, but usually only three or four. During the latent period the disease is not nearly as contagious as in the primary and secondary stages.

After so long a time, but sooner or later, the signs of late or tertiary syphilis appear, and in this stage literally every organ and part of the body can be affected. Frequent sites are the heart, blood vessels, brain, spinal cord, and bones, but syphilis is always considered a possible cause in the differential diagnosis of almost every serious disease of the human body. At this stage treatment can only prevent further advance and contagion of the disease, for irreversible organ damage has usually already occurred.

In pregnancy, syphilis carries a tremendous risk to the baby for the causal germ crosses the placenta into the body of the unborn child. Prior to the development of effective treatment methods, syphilis was the most common cause of stillbirth and premature delivery. It can also cause late miscarriage. Furthermore, numerous malformations of the baby can result from this infection. Even if these do not occur, the infant inherits the disease and will later develop the lesions of secondary and late syphilis.

With proper treatment of infected individuals and public health requirements of reporting the disease so that all sexual contacts can also be treated, the incidence of the disease has dropped 80 percent from its 1950 peak. Still we have about 25,000 new cases reported in the United States each year, and probably another 100,000 cases that are not reported. At present the incidence is on the increase but regular checkups with blood tests for syphilis can prevent *you* from falling prey to this predatory pestilence.

GONORRHEA (Clap)

At the present time, gonorrhea is the second most prevalent disease in the United States; only the common cold is more frequent. U.S. Health Department figures suggest that about one out of every one hundred young people is afflicted with this disease. Other studies indicate that 80 percent of women who have this disease are without symptoms but may become symptomatic at any time. The asymptomatic male is less common. For those of sexually liberated orientation, there is a definite hazard of exposure to this condition. You cannot tell from the way one is dressed or the apparent health of his physique whether or not he is afflicted. One helpful hint, however (used by most prostitutes), is to milk the penis forward, and if a discharge of pus occurs, run for your life! Of course, do not confuse this with the *clear* precoital secretion that occurs in most men in their anticipated sexual encounter.

Symptomatically, gonorrhea begins with a greenish-yellow, vaginal discharge which is not irritating. Then, usually following or during the next menstrual period, severe lower-abdominal pains and high fever (up to 106°) may occur. This is due to the upward spread of the bacteria through the womb into the fallopian tubes. Unless treated, spread to the ovaries occurs, and massive abscesses of the tubes and ovaries result. Pelvic peritonitis is also usual with such involvement. Needless to say, such degree of diseased damage to a woman usually causes permanent sterility. The peritonitis may even spread to the upper abdomen producing the so-called "violin string adhesions" around the liver. To be sure, this is no minor condition.

Further complications of gonorrhea include blood poisoning, infection of the inside of the heart, and even arthritis. In addition to the above, usual manifestations of this disease, infection and abscesses of the glands around the vagina and urethra may occur. Anal and oral infections are common if these areas are used for sexual recreation.

Fortunately, we now have antibiotic drugs that will cure this disease and constant vigilance, periodic checkups, and cultures for the causative germ can avoid its destructive disaster.

HERPES VIRUS DISEASE (H.V.D.)

H.V.D. is sometimes referred to as the new venereal disease as medical texts prior to 1965 rarely mentioned this infection. Basically there are two herpes virus organisms recognized—Type I, which usually occurs above the waist and produces the typical "fever blister," and Type II, which more commonly affects the genital area; however, neither type has a boundary limit, and either can cause infection in any area. Oral sexual activity is no doubt a factor in this infection. More common than syphilis, estimates indicate as many as 1,000,000 American women will have this disease in the next year.

Typically the symptoms of genital herpes show up five to seven days after exposure and cause a blistery lesion, very similar to a fever blister, which is very painful on the vulva. If the infection is in the vagina or cervix, few or no symptoms may occur. Although the lesion is usually singular, one-half to three-fourths inch in size, multiple lesions do occur. Needless to say, all sexual activity should be abandoned until the lesion heals. In the quiescent stage, contagion is unlikely.

Usually the sores will disappear in two to four weeks but tend to recur periodically. At the present writing there is no cure for this disease, although vaccines similar to smallpox have been used with good results in Germany.

Recent studies indicate a significant increase in the incidence of cancer of the cervix in infected women.

The most serious complication of H.V.D. occurs during pregnancy when the baby can contract the disease during delivery, and systemic infection in the newborn is usually fatal. For this reason most obstetricians prefer to deliver infected patients by Caesarean section in order to prevent the contamination of of the baby. Another relatively common viral infection, cytomegalovirus (C.M.V.), is considered a significant cause of malformations in the newborn. As this virus can be identified in the vagina or cervix of women and in the semen of males, its venereal significance is obvious.

CONDYLOMATA ACUMINATA (Venereal warts)

A common viral infection, unquestionably of venereal origin, genital warts are becoming more and more prevalent. It has long been known that they are more common during pregnancy and frequently go away after delivery. Probably the hormonal changes of pregnancy are conducive to this condition. By simulating the hormonal conditions of pregnancy with birth control pills, we have probably thereby increased the susceptibility and incidence of this disease.

Sometimes the warty growths on the vulva or perianal area may be singular, but usually they are multiple and may cover the entire vulva and vagina, even to the extent of massive cauliflower growths involving the entire labia or perianal area.

In the early stages these warts can be treated by a chemical, podophyllin, but in more advanced stages electrodessication, surgical excision, or freezing is necessary. A change in boyfriends may even be in order.

CHANCROID

Commonly referred to as "soft chancre," this disease is frequently confused with syphilis, which produces primarily a hard chancre. Chancroid is caused by a specific bacterium, *Hemophilus Ducreyi*. Much less common than the above infections, its venereal transmission is unquestioned. Last year only 1,200 cases were reported in the United States and most of these were males, but they probably got it from women who may have had no symptoms of the disease.

Generally in women the incubation period is considered

one to five days. The ulcerative, soft, painful lesion may occur on the labia, clitoris, around or even in the vagina, or on the anus. The ulcer is usually more irregular in shape, more tender, and softer than the chancre of syphilis, but special studies are necessary to differentiate between the two. About half the infected women will develop enlarged lymph nodes in the groin (buboes), which may be on one side only. Sometimes these lymph nodes develop into boils that may break open and drain spontaneously.

Fortunately we now have antibiotics which are very effective against this infection.

LYMPHOGRANULOMA VENEREUM (L.G.V.)

This is fortunately a rare disease (less than 600 cases per year in the United States) and most of these (99-plus percent) occur in blacks. However, the modern trend toward integrated sexual activity opens a new avenue of multiracial transmission. Its cause is a virus similar to the one that causes parrot fever. The incubation period is one to three weeks and the infection begins with a small, sometimes insignificant, lesion on the vulva, but soon an ulcerative drainage of the inguinal lymph nodes occurs. Sometimes elephantiastic enlargement of the vulva occurs. Probably through transmission by anal intercourse, the virus can cause such strictures of the rectum that obstruction of the bowel occurs, sometimes necessitating colostomy (an operation which opens the bowel through the abdominal wall).

In its early stages it can be treated, but unfortunately too many patients with this disease wait until the damage is irreversible.

GRANULOMA INGUINALE

Probably less contagious than lymphogranuloma venereum, the venereal nature of this infection is probable. It is caused by a bacterium, but fortunately it is rather rare, with less than one hundred cases reported in the United States last year. It is usually associated with other venereal diseases which confuse its diagnosis. In women it causes granulomatous lesions on the vulva, vagina, and enlarged, inguinal lymph nodes that can ulcerate and cause extensive destruction.

Once again, we now have antibiotics that can cure this condition.

CHLAMYDIA (Trachomatis)

This disease is usually asymptomatic in women but is a common cause of nongonorrheal urethritis in men. Some studies show as high as 8 percent of women harbor the organism which is midway between viruses and bacteria. The sexual transmission is unquestioned, and treatment of conjugal contacts is essential to eradicate the disease. Its main danger is the causation of serious eye infections in the newborn infants of infected mothers. However, recognition and prompt treatment can prevent permanent eye damage.

Although not generally considered venereal diseases, scabies, infectious hepatitis, infectious mononucleosis, molluscum contagiosum, and many other contagious diseases can be and are transmitted either through sexual intercourse or the close approximation of the human bodies in even petting practices.

PRURITUS VULVAE

Pruritus vulvae is by far the most froquent condition a gynecologist sees. Let me say at the outset that the various products advertised in newspapers and magazines for this problem are completely worthless, ineffectual, and may in themselves cause chemical or allergic inflammations. Usually they contain a local anesthetic agent which merely numbs the area, thus giving a false sense of improvement. Actually this only delays the proper diagnosis and treatment of the trouble. Incidentally a few drinks of liquor or dilute wine applied locally will temporarily ease itching, but it also won't cure anything.

All cases of pruritus have a cause, and before even the most learned physician can treat one effectively, he must *first* determine the cause. Sometimes it is very difficult to determine, but with careful study and perseverance the cause can almost always be found.

As a guide to women afflicted with pruritus let me offer some helpful suggestions:

(1) Do not try to treat the condition yourself or follow the advice of "friends" who may know even less than you do about it. (I once saw a patient who was advised by a "friend" to use turpentine. It took me a week to treat the chemical reaction to the turpentine before I could even start to diagnose the original condition.)

(2) Do not take a douche or use contraceptive foam or gel, or any other vaginal medication for several days before seeing the doctor.

(3) Do not be reluctant to tell the doctor of your personal hygiene and sexual habits so that he is not handicapped in his diagnostic evaluation of your problem.

(4) See a competent doctor as soon as possible after symptoms appear. These considerations will assure you of the speediest, most complete recovery.

The symptoms of pruritus are few in number but the causes may be numerous. Burning, itching, and irritation, with or without an abnormal discharge, are the cardinal signs. There can also be an abnormal discharge without irritation. The symptoms are only general and do not spell out any one particular disease. Only proper examination, including microscopic examination of the discharge, can pinpoint the cause of the condition. Because of the frequency of pruritus, however, I feel that every woman should know something about it—thus this discussion.

Twenty years ago fungus infections of the vagina (*Candida*

albicans) were considered rare. Now this is the most common vaginal infection seen in women. Essentially there are two reasons for this. First, there is widespread and frequently injudicious use of antibiotics which kill the lactobacillus—the guardian angel of the vagina. For instance, many patients receive, frequently at their own insistence, penicillin shots for a cold—a treatment proven beyond any possible doubt to be worthless. A week or ten days later, they experience a profuse discharge from the vagina, sometimes watery or sometimes of the consistency of cottage cheese. There is associated intense itching, swelling, redness of the vulva and vagina, and a burning pain on intercourse. Believe me, this condition is much more annoying than the cold—the injudicious treatment of which resulted in the fungus infection of the vagina by killing the lactobacillus and thereby making a fertile ground for harmful fungus germs. About 10 percent of the women who take a broad-spectrum antibiotic will develop a vaginal fungus infection.

Once the infection is acquired it is contagious and will promptly be transmitted to the partner. Men may have few or no symptoms. Sometimes they develop a rash on the penis, but usually they do not. There may be only a hypersensitivity of the glans penis. The fungus is harbored then by the male, and unless he is treated simultaneously with his wife, she will have a reinfection after treatment—the so-called Ping-Pong effect.

In addition to infection of the vagina, fungus infection of the mouth and intestinal tract can occur after antibiotic therapy. I once saw a woman who had an irritating discharge, irritation of the mouth, and mucus diarrhea. On further inquiry, I learned that a doctor had prescribed for her son some capsules that cost fifty cents each. She felt that any medicine that cost that much must be good, so she took two of them. On examination I found fungus infection of the mouth, the bowel, and the vagina—a dear price to pay for a capricious experiment in materia medica.

Since the mouth as well as the genitals (two areas frequently approximated in lovemaking) may be readily infected with the fungus and since the germ infestation may appear before symptoms occur, it is frequently indicated to treat both the genital areas of the male and female and their mouths as well.

The second factor in the prevalence of fungal infection of the vagina is birth control pills. It has long been known that pregnant women are very susceptible to fungus infections of the vagina due to the increased vascularity and secretions of lower acidity. In simulating the hormonal conditions of pregnancy, the birth control pills cause the same changes in the vagina that make it more susceptible to fungus infection. And in some cases with persistent and intractible infections of the vagina, I have had to discontinue prescribing birth control pills in favor of other contraceptive measures.

It is common to encounter fungus infections in women who have been to the beach. This is not so much due to the prevalence of these germs in the beach area, but rather the conduct of the women at such resorts. It is usually customary for them to put on a bathing suit in the morning and live in it all day. A bathing suit with its airtight crotch, the heat of the noonday sun, and the perspiration of the pent-up area is conducive to fungus infections, not to mention the increased and sometimes errant sexual activity occurring at these resorts.

For the beach enthusiast I recommend loose shorts with cotton underwear, or none, and the donning of a bathing suit only for swimming purposes. Even then the bathing suit should be adequately aired after use and the crotch turned inside out so that adequate air and sunshine can dry it thoroughly. Fungus can hardly survive such exposure.

Another predisposing factor in the causation of fungus infections is diabetes. Sometimes the first sign of diabetes will be monilia, which thrives on sugar. Thus any woman with fungus disease of the vulva, particularly if recurrent, should be checked for diabetes. Furthermore, the proper and adequate control of her diabetic condition will best protect her against persistent and recurrent infection.

TRICHOMONAS VAGINITIS (T.V.)

Although not generally considered to be a veneral disease, let me assure you that the sexual transmission of this disease is more frequent than that of syphilis. Second most common as a cause of pruritus, some estimates suggest as many as 20 percent of American women have this disease.

Symptomatically, T.V. produces a greenish-yellow, frothy, very foul discharge. In its acute stages, intense itching and ulceration of the vulva and vagina occur. The small ulcerations of the cervix produce the characteristic "strawberry" appearance. The cause is *Trichomonas vaginalis*, a small one-celled animal about the size of a white blood cell. Ordinarily this organism does not survive in the environment of the mouth or the rectum; thus its transmission is essentially by vaginal intercourse. In the male, the parasite can dwell in the urethra, seminal vesicles, and prostate gland, and is probably a common cause of male prostatitis.

In the untreated female the condition becomes chronic, but the profuseness and foulness of the discharge may abate, so that she is virtually asymptomatic. However, from time to time, the symptoms may spontaneously recur and seemingly a new infection has occurred.

Fortunately, we now understand the venereal nature of this disease. One drug (Metronidazole) will cure it if all sexual contacts are simultaneously treated. Unfortunately, alcohol sometimes reacts adversely with this drug so all forms of it should be avoided during the treatment period. There is some evidence that this infection may be associated with an increased incidence of cancer of the cervix.

It is quite ridiculous to try to mask the odor of this infection with perfumes, to combat its itching with anesthetic ointments, and to vitiate its discharge with douches. If you have problems, see a doctor.

BACTERIAL VAGINITIS

Most commonly, bacterial vaginitis is due to *Hemophilus vaginalis,* but occasionally we encounter other bacteria such as streptococci and staphylococci. I have even seen two cases of diphtheria of the vagina. (I leave the cause of this to your imagination.)

Typically, the bacterial infections of the vagina produce a foul, usually nonirritating, grayish, sometimes frothy, discharge and may or may not be sexually transmitted, but usually are. Thus simultaneous treatment of the male with appropriate antibiotics is essential in the management of this as well as all other forms of V.D. and pruritus.

PEDICULOSIS PUBIS (Crab lice, Phthirus pubis)

Traditionally, "crabs" have been considered a social stigma associated with vulgarity, promiscuity, and general filth and uncleanliness. Today in our permissive society, however, there are no class or sociological barriers to this disease. Fortunately, it is rather rare, but seems to be increasing. Although generally infection in adults is due to sexual intercourse, the organisms can be contracted from mutual bedding, toilet seats, and other nonsexual means. I have heard some people say facetiously that Texas crabs can jump ten feet!

The main symptom of crabs is itching, followed by excoriations and pustules in the pubic hair area. Usually the disease is localized in the pubic area, but can also infest the armpits, eyebrows, and even the head hair. Close inspection will reveal the tiny little animals which are somewhat smaller than a pinhead.

It is not necessary to shave the area for treatment, although I have seen many patients who did this on their own before consulting a physician. In addition to shaving, patients will frequently apply various "home remedies" such as blue ointment, bug sprays, and turpentine—all of which can cause severe chemical irritation, thus compounding the problem. Kwell lotion applied every night for about three nights will usually cure the infestation; however, it is important in order to avoid reinfection that the causative factors be eradicated. Particularly if contacted by sexual association, the partner must also be treated.

ALLERGIC REACTIONS

Allergic reactions can occur with all sorts of contraceptive methods and "feminine hygiene" products. With birth control pills, generalized skin rashes or hives can occur, but fortunately this type of reaction is quite rare. Allergic reactions to rubber condoms and diaphragms are more common than generally realized. Contraceptive creams and foams also take their toll in allergic reactions. Douche preparations, suppositories, foams, and for that matter, any medicinal or chemical substance put into the vagina can, in a sensitive person, produce an allergic reaction. In sensitized individuals the reaction may not be confined to the local vaginal-genital area but can even be quite generalized.

It is not uncommon for women to have allergic reactions to vaginal medications, and this can confuse the picture of vaginal irritation considerably. Recently I saw a patient who was diagnosed by another doctor as having a fungus infection. He had prescribed an appropriate medicine, and after two weeks of its use, she was seemingly unimproved because intense itching and swelling were still present; therefore the doctor referred her to me. On examination all I could see was a vagina full of medicine which she was using twice daily. She was rather upset when I told her I would prescribe no further treatment until a revaluation of her problem could be made. I told her to return in three days without any further medication or douches. When she returned she said, "I'm well." In retrospect, I'm sure she had a fungus infection which was properly treated. But she was allergic to the medicine, and although it had cured the fungus, it was causing a similar irritation. Continuation of treatment with a drug to which she was allergic would only have perpetuated her trouble.

This same type of perpetual vaginal irritation I have encountered frequently with douches, wherein the woman takes a douche and has allergic or even chemical irritation from the solution. Because of the irritation she takes another douche and another and another, never realizing that it is the douche itself that is the whole problem. The same situation can be caused by so-called "cleansing" suppositories.

In the sleuthing approach to uncover the cause of allergic reactions, I have sometimes detected them to be due to such seemingly innocuous agents as the perfumes and dyes in toilet paper. These ridiculous innovations just reemphasize the extent to which manufacturers will go to peddle their products, and in the highly competitive merchandising world it is hard to find plain white, nonscented toilet paper! Even the residue left in panties from laundry products can produce chemical or allergic irritations.

Bubble baths can cause allergic reactions, too—not only for you, but for little girls, as well.

If you're using toiletries, cosmetics, and so forth that cause you no irritation, stick to them. If the urge to experiment overtakes you, try a new product, but discontinue it at once if the reaction is bad. You might end up a victim rather than a vamp.

A recent letter from a grateful patient explains far better than I can the pertinence of these admonitions:

Dear Dr. Busby,

Regarding my somewhat impromptu visit to your office in late December—I appreciated very much your accepting me as a patient again. The vaginal irritation cleared up many weeks ago as a result of permitting my body the freedom of no underwear at night, reduced usage of synthetic underclothes, and a taboo on perfumes and perfumed soap.

So, having resigned myself to the wearing of drab cotton underwear and no perfume, I appear less sexy but much more comfortable!

Many thanks!

CHAPTER 7

Heads and Tails

IT is perhaps symbolic that usually when a coin is flipped, the caller asks for heads, but occasionally one wins with tails. Whether or not this has some deep subconscious Freudian significance or not I don't know, but it is interesting to speculate that it may be an "id" indication of sexual preference. It has long been colloquial to refer to coital activity as "a piece of tail." Nevertheless, to each his own.

It is not my purpose to describe or otherwise present the erotic sensations imparted by oral or anal sex. Those who have already indulged are familiar with those pleasures; but for those who haven't, they could open the door to a new wonderland of sensuous delectation! Such books as *The Sensuous Woman, The Joy of Sex,* and numerous other publications have already exploited those aspects. My thoughts deal only with the medical aspects from the standpoint of health and disease. According to the Kinsey report, oral sex is more common among educated people than among know-nots. Perhaps this is due to fewer hang-ups from the taboos of ignorance. Frequently I refer to it as the Kinsey I.Q. test. The more recent *Playboy* survey indicates about 85 percent of people indulge in oral activity, and of the younger generation, about 25 percent are having anal sex, but my own professional experience suggests this figure is somewhat on the low side.

For the uninitiated, oral sex consists of cunnilingus (muff diving, giving head, eating out), and fellatio (blow job, plating, giving head, sucking off). Unfortunately these fun practices have some hazards of which most participants are unaware. For the normal, healthy person they are perfectly safe, but when disease is present, another avenue of transmission is opened. For instance, fungus infection of the vagina can be transmitted to the penis and to the mouth. This form of infection is not uncommon in the newborn of a mother with this infection. As the baby passes through the birth canal, it acquires the infection in his mouth. This form is commonly called thrush, but the causative organism is the same. In the adult the infection may produce white plaques in the mouth with redness, swelling, and soreness. Although the woman may have been adequately and properly treated for the vaginal infection, failure to treat the mouths of all parties concerned will most assuredly be a source of reinfection. I have encountered a number of cases in which, probably due to the naïveté of the doctor rather than lack of knowledge, failure of treatment occurred.

A case in point was a couple I had known for many years who had moved to another city. The couple approached me at a cocktail party one evening and told me that they had been treated for two years by a gynecologist for a persistent fungus infection. I knew the doctor to be a very competent and able man. I told this pair that if they would come to my office the next day, I would do what I could for them. (Cocktail-party advice from doctors is usually no better than from lay people. I have always said, "Free advice is worthless.") When they arrived, I asked the husband to step into my examining room. He immediatcly started to remove his pants, but instead I told him to open his mouth. A smear of his saliva was positive for fungus. He stated that the doctor had treated his wife and his penis, but not his mouth. I prescribed appropriate measures and I have seen this couple periodically since that time without evidence of recurrence. This incident confirms an age-old teaching in medicine that more mistakes are made from not looking than from not knowing.

Unfortunately patients are usually reluctant to divulge their sexual practices, a handicap to the doctor in both diagnosis and treatment. A more candid approach by the patient would assure her of better medical care. On several occasions I have been rebuked by holier-than-thou Victorian prudes when I merely asked if they were having oral sex. Over the years I have learned to presume that everyone is doing it and treat patients accordingly without explaining the reasoning behind my somewhat unorthodox treatment.

Surely by now most people know that syphilis can be transmitted by kissing as well as by other affectionate gestures, but few people realize that gonorrhea can be transmitted this way. To be sure, gonorrheal tonsillitis and pharyngitis can and do occur. Actually, innumerable diseases are transmitted by oral sexual contacts and some almost exclusively this way. For example, Vincent's infection which causes an acute, necrotic ulceration with foul, purulent drainage is the same disease as "trench mouth." The new common herpes viral infection of the vulva is frequently associated with oral sex. In many cases of venereal warts (condylomata acuminata), a disease generally considered to be caused by a virus, the male partner has no warts on his penis. Probably the method of transmission is by oral contact. It is also interesting that the common vaginal infection, trichomoniasis, does not usually occur in the mouth. As the brain is the most sensuous sexual organ in the body, the mouth is the most dangerous from the standpoint of transmission of disease.

Just be careful. Don't fellate on the first date!

PSYCHOSEMENALYSIS

The reactions of women to semen are myriad. To some it is as revolting as the slimy trail of the snail; but to the connoisseur, it is more like the delicacy, escargots. In between are those who can take it or leave it, neither being turned on or off by it, almost as if it were completely inorganic. On the other hand, many women are completely fascinated with the process of ejaculation —love to watch it occur, love to feel its eruption, love to play with it, love to rub it into their skin (for which it has been inappropriately accredited with having multiple benefits), and even love to taste it. Whatever your pleasure, it's all normal. As an example, however, of abnormal reaction to this harmless substance, I once had a patient who had had a complete hysterectomy but would not let her husband have intercourse with her without using a rubber condom, lest the semen should touch her vagina. Naturally she was childless. Clearly her viewpoint was psychopathologic, undoubtedly resulting from a super-Victorian warning beyond the realm of reason.

Chemically the composition of semen varies considerably from individual to individual, and from time to time with the same individual. Its volume and consistency vary with the health of the man, his frequency of ejaculation, and even the duration of foreplay, or anticipation of the sexual encounter. About 92 percent of semen is water, the rest contains fructose (fruit sugar), ascorbic acid (as in lemon juice), cholesterol (not enough to interfere with your diet, if you're on low cholesterol), creatine, pyruvic acid, glutathrone, lactic acid (an ingredient of milk), urea, uric acid, vitamin B–12, various salts such as sodium, potassium, phosphorus, ammonia, magnesium, and a variety of enzymes and hormones such as testosterone, estrogen, and prostaglandins. But in any event, none of these substances are harmful in any way and the swallowing of semen can cause no bodily harm, nor can it cause any form of pregnancy, a question I am asked frequently! It contains only three to five calories, and although otherwise may be considered nutritious, it is certainly not fattening!

In my experience the vast majority of women who carry fellatio to completion do swallow the semen, and some even experience orgasm from doing so. Actually most men feel rejected when a woman, on completion of this act, gags, retches or vomits —so if you're going to fellate, consummate!

It is rather interesting in this connection to note that most "Johns" of prostitutes are married men who seek sexual releases not granted at home and, of course, most frequent of these is fellatio! Any woman sufficiently motivated, without hang-ups, with sufficient practice, can do this as well as any hooker. This is a frequent hang-up between married couples (as well as anal intercourse) that can and sometimes does cause a marriage to end in divorce. If your heart (more anatomically correct, your mouth) isn't in it, then don't do it just because you're trying to salvage an otherwise doomed marriage. With sex, as in all other human relationships, you are never too old to learn, and hopefully my comments may relieve any tensions you may have in this regard.

ANAL INTERCOURSE

If you are not interested in this subject, please skip the remainder of this chapter. If you haven't tried it, don't knock it; but if you're on the fence, let me give you some pros and cons. Although commonly referred to as dirty and base, it is interesting to note that Freud said fourscore years ago that obstinacy, stinginess, and *orderliness* are the personality traits that are traceable to anal erotism. Although I am quite familiar with reports from large proctologic clinics in New York and other metropolitan areas which include unusual and bizarre problems from such encounters, my own experience with patients (numbering in the hundreds) whom I know practice this with some degree of regularity, do not experience any ill effects. In the large clinics which deal with colo-proctologic disease, the usual patient presents himself because of a disease or pathologic problem. To be sure I have seen the reports of extreme injury of the rectum, X-ray pictures of Coca-Cola bottles, light bulbs, and other foreign bodies lodged in the rectum, the lacerations and infections associated with anal eroticism. The clinics' anti-anal viewpoints are really based more on disease that may or may not be a result of this practice or, at least, a deviant degree of same beyond the customary (and normal) considerations of this communication. I do not know if it is cause or effect, but in my experience with women who occasionally or even frequently practice this method of sexual expression, I have never seen one who suffered from hemorrhoids, fissures, or even constipation. It is interesting in this respect to note that in the surgical treatment of both anal fissures and hemorrhoids, dilation of the anal sphincter is basic. This comment should not necessarily be construed to mean that this practice is therapeutic, but it is common in the United States to treat minor fissures of the anus with dilations, and recent reports from England show high success rates with treating hemorrhoids by rectal dilations alone.

As stated earlier, few people are born with the problem of constipation; this is almost always an acquired personality quirk. Perhaps the most important contributory factor in women is the postponement of the defecatory urge, which is no more abnormal than hunger or thirst. By so doing, they accomplish, over the years, a spasm of the anal sphincter in order to prevent the fulfillment of this natural (and frequently enjoyable) function of the human body. In time this produces what I call "tight-ass syndrome," a persistent spasm of the sphincteric musculature which impairs its normal function in being able to relax for one's natural elimination, and by its very spasm is actually conducive to the development of hemorrhoids and fissures.

In cases of "tight-ass syndrome," the passage of any but small, soft stools can cause tearing of the anal mucosa—to wit, a fissure. Also people with this condition who strain to defecate can cause protrusion of a dilated hemorrhoidal blood vessel and the tight sphincter contracts violently against it preventing return of the inspissated blood so that thrombosis (blood clot) with its accompanying pain and protrusive projection can occur. Whether or not you choose to have anal intercourse is really a matter of personal preference and ideological concepts, but you can still avoid the potentially hazardous condition of "tight-ass syndrome" by always yielding to the natural urge for your bowels to move, which is just as American as apple pie.

Another large factor in the problem of constipation is lack of fluid intake. Actually most constipation is really only a matter of dehydration of the stool. The colon and rectum are capable of absorbing water from the intestinal debris, and by so doing, the stool left in the colon can become hard, firm, and inflexible. In the straining efforts to pass such a bolus, lacerations (fissures) of the anal mucosa and protrusions of hemorrhoidal vessels, dilated by the very straining itself, can result.

Actually, the anal area is richly supplied with sensory nerves and is generally considered one of the erogenous zones. Most women (and men too, for that matter) derive considerable sexual arousal from tactile, oral, or penetrative stimulation of this area. On the other hand, some people respond negatively to the idea of anal intercourse—a taboo augmented by the sodomy laws of most states, probably enacted by solons who were doing it themselves.

Some women report a painful reaction to anal intercourse; however, if one considers that even the most pleasurable sensations of orgasm are neurologically transmitted by pain nerve fibers, it is understandable that even the pain can intensify the sensuous response for some people. As is commonly commented concerning vaginal intercourse, "It hurts so good!" In my experience with women who indulge in this form of eroticism, the reactions vary widely. Some definitely don't like it; some tolerate it as a benevolence to their lovers; some say they enjoy it immensely, even to the point of having quicker and more intense orgasms in this manner; and a few even prefer it to vaginal intercourse.

Nevertheless, a few precautionary parables do apply to this activity. First of all, the anus (and rectum) has no secretory glands like the vagina, therefore artificial lubrication is necessary. Saliva or vaginal secretions (unless copious) are inadequate for this encounter. Also surgical lubricants such as K-Y Jelly are water emulsions and tend to dry out leaving an undue friction on a sensitive and vulnerable area, thus a more lasting lubrication such as petroleum jelly (Vaseline) or butter is much more satisfactory. For the anal virgin, dilation of the sphincter muscle with one or two fingers will facilitate insertion of the penis and markedly reduce any pain produced by this. It is generally advised by medical authorities not to insert the penis in the rectum and then into the vagina, lest infection should occur. Actually infection of the vagina due to the bacteria normally found in the lower bowel, is practically unknown. Even in patients who suffer from recto-vaginal fistulae (holes between the vagina and the rectum) as a result of childbirth injuries, or from radiation treatment of cancer where the vagina is constantly under the bacteriological barrage of fecal contents, infection does not usually ensue. Also in obstetrical delivery, lacerations of the anus into the vagina are not uncommon, where spillage of the fecal material is unavoidable, yet infection is so unusual that most obstetricians do not even administer antibiotics under these circumstances. Nevertheless, as a matter of simple hygiene and aesthetics, it would usually be advisable to wash the penis after an anal encounter before proceeding to vaginal intercourse.

ANILINGUS

As an extension of cunnilingus, as a prelude to anal intercourse, or as a stimulating practice in itself (both to the anilingee and the anilingor) this practice is probably more common than would ordinarily be suspected. But even though in practice it may be relatively infrequent, its vernacular invitation is probably one of our most common epithets. As mentioned above, the anal area in most people is highly erogenous and tactile or particularly oral stimulation of this region is especially titillating! With proper cleansing prior to such an encounter, this should not be considered unaesthetic; however, there are some disease hazards, probably more so from the mouth side than the anal side! Normally the vulva is covered by the colon bacillus, and this is not related to which way the female wipes after defecating, but rather because this is a motile bacterium and can migrate on its own accord. Also, many other parasitic infections of the bowel have migratory ability, so that actually from a disease standpoint, anilingus is no more dangerous than cunnilingus. Both can be a source of all sorts of intestinal parasites such as pinworms, roundworms, tapeworms, amoeba, infectious hepatitis, tuberculosis, dysentery, as well as the more common venereal diseases. On the other hand, the mouth can impart to this area syphilis, gonorrhea, herpes virus and even venereal warts, so know your partner.

HUMAN BITES

Although a certain amount of licking, sucking, and nibbling is usual in sexual foreplay, if carried to the extreme of biting to the point of breaking skin, serious infection can occur. The human mouth carries a wide variety of disease-causing germs, but because of the mouth's relative immunity to them, there is usually no infection in the mouth, but infections can be imposed on almost any other part of the body by biting. Before the discovery of antibiotics, infections from human bites were sometimes fatal.

Even intense sucking of various parts of the body can produce bruises or "hickeys" which are painful and take several weeks to resolve.

Although intense sucking and biting are usually involuntary due to the loss of emotional control in the throes of passion, sometimes we find people, both men and women, who include such acts as routine in their sexual expressions. Unless you have masochistic leanings, avoid them.

CHAPTER 8

Dyspareunia Is No Petunia

DYSPAREUNIA (painful intercourse) is all too commonly a presenting complaint of female patients. The causes are numerous, at times multiple, and occasionally baffle the most learned physician. It has been said that dyspareunia is better than no pareunia, for regardless of its cause, pain on coitus does not necessarily preclude orgasm.

The physicial causes of this condition include many pelvic diseases such as endometriosis, uterine fibroids, ovarian cysts, pelvic infections, and vaginitis, particularly of the fungus variety. However, there are numerous other causes which can be categorized as psychologic, physiologic, or pathologic, that give the same symptom.

Endometriosis produces nodules in the pelvis which are as sore as boils, especially around the time of the menstrual period, and the persistent prodding of these areas with penile thrusting causes a real, and at times very severe, pain. As the possibility of slight internal bleeding can also occur, the pain may last several hours or even several days.

With uterine fibroids or ovarian cysts, the trauma to the affected parts can cause bruising, twisting, or swelling such as to exaggerate any pain that these conditions may normally cause. It is not uncommon for small ovarian cysts to actually be ruptured during coitus as the ovary may be impaled behind the vagina against the sacral bone. This event can give rise to considerable internal bleeding—a cause of severe pain, as blood is very irritating to the peritoneal cavity. Rarely this condition requires surgery to arrest the bleeding.

As to pelvic infection, there is usually pain present which is merely exacerbated by the act of intercourse. If the infection is limited to the vagina, particularly as a fungus, only a burning pain occurs. This burning may also occasionally be experienced by the male. In women past the menopause another form of vaginitis (senile or atrophic) occurs from hormone deficiency. This produces a rather raw texture to the vaginal surface and dryness from lack of secretion that can give rise to a penetrating pain such as encountered with putting salt on a cut.

Another frequently encountered, physical cause of dyspareunia is episiotomy scars. (Episiotomy is the cut made in the lower vagina to enlarge its opening for childbirth.) This is almost invariably due to the incision's being made obliquely to avoid the rectum, for dyspareunia following episiotomies done in the midline—toward the rectum—practically never cause this problem, even if extension or laceration into the rectum occurs. Fortunately, nowadays most obstetricians are well aware of this possible result, and now midline incisions are usually done.

Sometimes rectal conditions, because of their proximity to the vagina, can cause dyspareunia. These would include such common conditions as anal fissures, hemorrhoids, or even constipation.

Women who have undergone radium treatments for cancer of the womb and (rarely) women past the menopause acquire strictures of the vagina which make intercourse painful or even impossible. I have even encountered a case where the persistent use of overly strong Lysol douches scarred and constricted the vagina to such an extent that even a pencil could not be inserted into it.

Whenever clear-cut pelvic disease which accounts for the causation of dysparenuia is found, the problem is relatively simple, for institution of appropriate medical or surgical treatment will usually relieve it. On the other hand, the vast majority of cases of dyspareunia is completely normal on physical and laboratory examinations; thus the plot deepens.

One of the most common causes of dyspareunia is inadequate lubrication. This is more frequent among married couples, where there is a tendency to shortcuts, inadequate foreplay, and lack of sufficient prestimulation of the woman to provoke the natural secretions of arousal. This tendency to dryness is physiologically augmented in women after the menopause and sometimes in young women on birth control pills. Although a common condition, its treatment is amazingly simple. I generally advise couples that if they don't have at least two hours to make love, not to start! Although it might not take that long, at least one doesn't feel the need to punch the time clock in five minutes! There are no World Fair grand prizes or Olympic medals given to the winner of a "Wham-bang, thank you ma'am" contest! From a practical standpoint, the most effective way to overcome the dyspareunic problem of excessive dryness is by the direct application of saliva—not only is it lubricating, but the very mechanism of its direct application will usually provoke a simultaneous response of vulvovaginal secretion which will obtain the desired objective.

There are other physiological causes of painful intercourse which can be related to a woman's menstrual cycle. At the time of ovulation there can be a small amount of internal bleeding which will cause pain that will be worsened by intercourse. Also some women, because of the pelvic congestion that occurs as the period approaches, may experience pain on intercourse at this time.

Another common cause of dyspareunia and postcoital pain is orgasmic failure. All men are familiar with the condition of "hot nuts" produced by unfulfilled sexual excitation, but most are unknowledgeable that a similar condition occurs in women. In the state of sexual stimulation, the woman undergoes a state of pelvic congestion—an engorgement of the pelvic organs with blood, a condition called tumescence. Following orgasm a state of detumescence occurs wherein not only is the sexual urge satisfied but the engorgement of the pelvic viscera is also relieved. If not relieved, this can cause true pelvic pain which can last for several hours or even a day, possibly more. As the male with "hot nuts" attempts to relieve his problem by masturbating, the best relief for a woman is the same, to give her sexual release and thereby accomplish the desired state of detumescence. What a pity! But in keeping with modern concepts it is better to do one's own thing than nothing! It's better than pain pills, ill-advised operations, or suffering—be it physical or mental.

Frigidity, impotence, and dysparenuia are all closely related, both physically and psychologically. When one loses interest in sex, it can be a psychologically painful experience, regardless of the cause of the lack of interest. Some chronic and debilitating diseases such as diabetes, cancer, tuberculosis, and mental disease —particularly depression—can cause sexual inadequacy. Sometimes it may merely be due to loss of interest in one's partner. Not only do they experience pain on intercourse, but also on discourse, the golf course, or any other activity they may engage in together. These are among the most difficult cases to solve because neither party will admit to any fault, deficiency, or lack of attentiveness. On careful inquiry I have found many women who complained of dyspareunia with their husbands but not with their lovers. Furthermore, this is not related to penis size, for frequently one finds the painless partner has the larger organ.

The psychological causes of painful intercourse are probably more numerous than the number of positions for having intercourse. Frequently the die is cast in early childhood by the attitudes imposed on the child by parents. "Don't touch yourself there." "This spot is a no-no." "Bad girl." "Never let anyone touch you there." These are common admonitions of overly Victorian parents who instill into the child a lifelong revulsion to the most pleasurable part of the body. Sometimes it takes years on the psychiatrist's couch to change this distorted viewpoint—and unfortunately in some cases it can never be overcome. This same kind of upbringing can also cause frigidity and fear of intercourse. As an example, I was recently consulted by a woman in her mid-thirties who had been married for twelve years. She said her marriage was about to crumble and she needed help. After some lengthy questioning I found that because of her childhood discipline she had never undressed in front of her husband and had only had intercourse with the lights out, under the covers, and in the "missionary" position—for twelve years! As a matter of fact, I have known many couples who have spent their entire marital lifetime with such restrictions and inhibitions.

There is no question that these patients need help badly, but to overcome such a background takes a long time, compassionate understanding, and a dedicated determination to remedy the problem. Although it is completely illogical, these women (and many men, for that matter) believe that restriction of sexual activity is more moral than pursuing a more varied approach to lovemaking. There are still many who believe that women are not supposed to be orgasmic and if they are, this is a sign of lewd baseness which is unbecoming and inappropriate for a "lady." Actually, I know of no religious or moral teaching that says sex is for men only and women are only supposed to indulge in it for the pleasure of men.

Other psychological causes of frigidity and dyspareunia include such experiences as child molestation, rape, incest, even improper or injudicious examinations or instrumentations by doctors, or the encountering of an exhibitionist. Sometimes observing one's parents making love is interpreted by a child as a form of brutality, or at least something that the observer would never want to do. Even teen-agers rarely can accept the fact that their parents engage in such activities, especially just for fun. Many children still believe (and have been encouraged in this idea by the pedestaled mother) that they were immaculately conceived. These girls do not masturbate and only superficially and disdainfully cleanse the vulval area. Why should they? They have been taught that this is a dirty area and should be maintained so!

Sometimes this type of background paves the way for a condition known as vaginismus (a spasm of the vaginal muscles). This condition can render intercourse not only painful but even impossible. Basically a panic reaction, vaginismus is very difficult to overcome, either with gynecologic or psychologic treatment—or both. I have encountered cases married for six months to two years who still suffer the consequences of this condition. Although with proper counseling these patients can learn to understand their problem, its causation and irrationality, they still cannot always overcome the reflexive spasms that occur whenever they attempt coitus. The word (of Momma) is mightier than the sword!

Occasionally one encounters painful intercourse (or frigidity) from simple physical revulsion toward the husband, because of B.O. from lack of cleanliness, beer breath or other forms of halitosis, or lack of grooming, shaving, etc. The husband is painful to see (or smell), let alone embrace. This form of dyspareunia only occurs with husbands, for singles will not tolerate this form of effrontery.

Fear of pregnancy is a frequent cause of coital pain and frigidity. This can be a very real threat to an otherwise compatible relationship. On the other side of the coin is the woman who loses interest in, or has pain from, sex after a sterilizing operation, or finds out from tests that she is unable to conceive. In the latter instance the woman feels that since no procreation is possible, the encounter is pointless.

Unfortunately, many physicians show no interest in patients' dyspareunic problems. As doctors are not mind readers, it is necessary for women to tell them the whole story about their difficulty. This should be done frankly and openly, just as if one were describing the symptoms of a cold. The doctor is then made aware of the condition and will examine more closely for possible causes. Frequently, all that is necessary to solve these problems is a little understanding, reassurance, and education of the patient. Although occasionally psychiatric or sexual therapy consultation is necessary, most interested physicians can resolve the majority of dyspareunic difficulties.

CHAPTER 9

To Be or Not to Be —Pregnant

IT seems that there are basically two types of woman—those who want to be, and those who do not want to be pregnant. At the present time, the latter group seems to be way ahead.

Although we think of contraception as a modern concept, it is interesting to note that in Soranus's *Gynecology* (ca. 100 A.D.) numerous methods of preventing pregnancy were described, such as pomegranate peel and oak gall suppositories, or drinking of cyrenaic balm, wallflower seed and myrtle in wine. These things were said not only to prevent conception, but were also considered abortifacients. Of course, today we know the complete ineffectiveness of such procedures, but it at least shows that attempts at contraception have been made for thousands of years.

"There is nothing perfect under the sun" appropriately applies even to modern contraception. Even though we have methods that are extremely effective, there are also some dangers in their use. As a matter of fact, it seems that the hazards are proportional to the relative effectiveness. At the present time approximately one woman in five thousand who becomes pregnant will die of some complication of pregnancy, a risk considerably greater than using any kind of contraception. Moreover, abortion, although now legal, is more dangerous than any type of preventive measure.

As no one method of contraception is suitable for all women, let us consider all the individual methods. Relative expense of these methods is hardly a consideration any more because family-planning clinics all over the country provide a variety of methods without charge. Nevertheless, if one compares the cost of having and rearing a child, all methods of contraception are extremely inexpensive.

ORAL CONTRACEPTIVES

It has long been known that superfetation (conception during an existing pregnancy) does not occur. The ovary does not produce eggs during pregnancy because of the inhibiting effect of the pregnancy hormones estrogen and progesterone. In this same inhibition of ovarian function by artificially administering these hormones which simulate pregnancy, not only does failure of ovulation occur, but many of the other symptoms of pregnancy are observed, such as nausea and vomiting, enlargement and/or secretion from the breasts, increased vascularity of the vagina and pelvic organs, fluid retention and weight gain, and chloasma (brownish area of discoloration of the skin, particularly on the forehead and face); for that matter, just about all the symptoms of early pregnancy can occur.

As to effectiveness, there is no question that the pill is the most effective method of contraceptive presently available, exceeding 99.7 percent. For some women pregnancy is a more undesirable event than for others; so if you're strongly desirous of the most effective method, then consider the pill. Certainly from an aesthetic standpoint the oral method is most appealing because no additional paraphernalia or mechanical contrivances are needed. One is always ready and safe.

Oral contraception has been used in the United States since 1960. It is now estimated that more than 10,000,000 women are on the pill. At present there are essentially two types of oral contraceptives: those containing a combination of estrogen and progesterone (hormones normally produced by the functioning ovary), and those that contain only progesterone. A third type containing only estrogen for the first fifteen of sixteen pills, and a mixture of estrogen and progesterone for five days (called sequentials), has been removed from the market. The combination products are more effective than the progestins alone. In addition to their efficacy as contraceptives, the combination pills also will ease most menstrual problems such as excessive and painful flow and irregularity. However, the Food and Drug Administration will not permit the manufacturers to advertise or recommend this advantage! As a matter of fact, combination pills have been used in the treatment of endometriosis.

As most of the dangerous side effects of oral contraceptives are due to the estrogen content, the progesterone alone pills have some advantages in safety for the woman, but they are not as effective for contraception, and unpredictable menstruation occurs. These variations may include spotting between periods (called breakthrough bleeding), prolonged or shortened duration of menstruation, and completely irregular periods. For those women who cannot tolerate, or have contraindications to estrogen, the progesterone pills should be considered. Different from the combination pills, which are taken intermittently, the progestin alone pill is taken continuously. This should not be confused with the popular packaging practice of making twenty-eight-day packs, the last seven of which are usually of a different color and contain no hormones but may contain iron. These last seven are just counters for women who cannot count to keep up with their cycles. I call these idiot packs. Who wants to take a blank pill every day for a week?

Oral contraceptives should never be taken by women who have had any form of thrombophlebitis, strokes, or pulmonary embolism (blood clots in the lungs). This does not include the mere presence of varicose veins. (Many women have the mistaken idea that varicose veins are a contraindication to the pill.)

Although as yet there is no evidence that the pill causes cancer, estrogen does stimulate the growth of many kinds of cancer, particularly of the breasts and pelvic organs. Those who have, or have had, cancer should not take oral contraceptives. Also, women with marked impairment of liver function, such as cirrhosis, should avoid this method.

Since abnormal uterine bleeding may be a sign of cancer, tumors, or pelvic infections, women with this problem should first have the cause of the abnormal bleeding determined before taking oral contraceptives.

All women taking the pill should have regular examinations —including Pap smears—at least every year, or better, every six months. Between visits to the doctor, the woman taking pills should be advised to report any swelling, soreness, or pain in the legs to him. Other danger signals may be a sudden pain in the chest with pain on deep breathing, loss or partial loss of vision, or other eye problems, and migraines.

Actually, true menstruation does not occur with the pill, but rather a periodic withdrawal bleeding, which simulates menstruation, takes place. Sometimes this may be little or even none, but since failures of oral contraceptives can happen rarely, it would be advisable for any woman who misses two periods on the pill to have a pregnancy test. Particularly those women who have missed taking one or more of their pills should consider the possibility of pregnancy even if just one period is missed.

As some of the hormones pass into the breast milk, nursing mothers should avoid the pill. Furthermore, the hormonal effect of the pill tends to dry up milk production.

Other undesirable side effects of oral contraception include increased size of uterine myomas (fibroids). As with cancer, there is no evidence that the hormones actually cause the fibroids, only that they can make them grow faster. At times mental changes—particularly depression—can occur. Also changes in libido—either increased or decreased—can result from the pill. Very rarely women, when stopping the pill, may have long periods of amenorrhea (loss of menstruation) and infertility. Usually this will spontaneously take care of itself after a few months, but it has been known to last for one or more years. Sometimes medical treatment of this condition is necessary.

A few words of caution to those taking the pills are in order. To be effective, the pills must be taken regularly whether or not intercourse takes place. If you miss or skip taking the pill, bleeding will probably occur and pregnancy can occur. For women who have difficulty swallowing any kind of pill, oral contraceptives may be an undue burden. For those who claim to have difficulty in remembering to take the pill, I recommend that they put a sign on the bathroom mirror or a tag on their toothbrush (it seems most women do remember to brush their teeth every day) that says, "Did you take your pill today?"

Contrary to popular belief that the pill must be taken at least a month before it is effective, the pills, if started on the fifth day of the menstrual period (the day the period *starts* is the first day), are effective immediately. If perchance you forget to take one or more pills, then other protection should be used. The pill, as with other methods of contraception, fails usually because of improper usage rather than the method itself!

The oral contraceptive method imparts a relaxed atmosphere of sexual expression as the fear of undesired pregnancy is relieved. To many women the fear of pregnancy can be a real hang-up, even to the point of complete frigidity. To such women the pill is a godsend and frequently may be instantly therapeutic.

Recent British studies suggest that women over forty may have an increased incidence of corony thrombotic heart disease from birth control pills (just another form of thrombotic disease). Although these reports have not been substantiated in this country, or elsewhere, the F.D.A. has already recommended that women over forty should not take birth control pills. They do not say what alternative precautions should be taken, only that some other method of birth control should be used!

The woman over forty is the one who has the greatest fear of pregnancy and rightly so, for in this age group the danger both to the mother and child is greatly increased. Moreover, the unwanted arrival of a "bundle from heaven" (or perhaps hell!) at this time of life can cause a massive domestic destruction. As a result, many women resort to major surgical procedures with their concomitant risks, sexually unsatisfactory methods of contraception, or fear frigidity—perhaps the worst consequence of all.

If a woman considers the problem in broad perspective, hopefully with the help of her family physician or gynecologist, then the solution for each individual case can be determined on its own merit rather than by the dictates of a domineering bureaucracy. Recently I have had many patients leave my office in a flood of tears when I informed them that the F.D.A. warns against the use of birth control pills for women over forty. It is indeed unfortunate that this governmental agency spreads only fear, trepidation, and uncertainty, rather than help, consolation, and comfort! Possibly their efforts will result in an epidemic of women over forty morosely pregnant, and the birth of numbers of subnormal children!

There is one other form of temporary oral contraception approved by the Federal Drug Administration and that is the "morning-after" pill. If begun on the day or two after unprotected exposure, but not after four days, diethylstilbesterol is particularly effective in preventing pregnancy. This method is especially helpful for rape victims. Actually, the "morning-after" pill is not really a contraceptive but an abortifacient. It does not prevent the connection of the egg and the sperm, but instead alters the lining of the womb (endometrium) by its hormonal effect, making it unreceptive for the implantation of the fertilized egg, a process that usually takes about eight days from the time of conception. Although this method exceeds 95 percent in effectiveness, it is not one which can be used frequently or repeatedly, for menstrual function is significantly altered by it and excessive use of diethylstilbesterol can cause serious flooding.

I.U.D.

As a contraceptive instrument, I.U.D. stands for intrauterine device, but from a more realistic perspective it could easily stand for "Invention Uv Devil"! Truly, this is the Edsel of modern contraceptive technology! I say "modern," but this is inappropriate for even in ancient times stones were placed in the wombs of camels to prevent pregnancy, as a pregnant camel was a poor pack animal. Even in the nineteenth century numerous intrauterine devices were introduced for the prevention of pregnancy and the induction of abortion. Since around 1924 many designs of devices and materials for their construction have been intensively investigated.

The earlier models such as the Grafenberg ring, the "collar button," and "wishbone" were made of various metals such as gold, silver, or stainless steel. Infection, abnormal bleeding, pain, and even uterine perforation were not uncommon complications of those earlier devices. The recently developed polyester plastic devices, which give little or no tissue reaction, can be inserted relatively easily through a very small inserter that usually does not require dilation of the cervix. As to efficacy, reports vary from 90 to 97 percent for different designs, but all are much less effective than oral contraceptives. Unfortunately we still have the problems of infection, abnormal bleeding, and uterine perforation, but not nearly so frequently as with the earlier metal devices.

It has been my custom to tell every patient in whom I

insert one of these instruments to expect every kind of bleeding known to man. Usually the abnormal bleeding occurs shortly after the insertion, but I have seen both bleeding between the periods and menstrual flooding begin several years after the insertion. I have even had to remove I.U.D.s in the middle of the night and at other inappropriate times because of massive flooding occuring years after the insertion. It is a natural effect for the muscular wall of the womb to rebel against any foreign body placed within it, and at times rather violent contractions occur and cramping pains ensue. These contractions may be sufficient to expel the device and this does occur in about 4 percent of insertions. Although usually the expulsion takes place within the early months of use, I have known them to be expelled years after insertion. Unfortunately, the woman is not always aware of the expulsion (a fact I have never been able to fathom), and one may not know it is gone until pregnancy results. The newer forms of I.U.D.s contain a small amount of barium so they can be identified by X ray, and they also have a small plastic thread which protrudes from the cervix into the vagina to facilitate removal of the device when desired. It is generally advised that women wearing I.U.D.s check this string every week by inserting the index finger well into the vagina. Unfortunately, many women cannot feel the strings at all and, of course, panic for fear that the I.U.D. has been expelled. Sometimes because the string is short or because the device has receded higher into the uterus, I cannot feel or even see the strings myself. Then it becomes necessary to take an X ray to see if the device is still in place. The protruding string provides a channel for bacteria to enter the womb, a situation ordinarily prevented by the thick mucous that fills the cervical canal. For this reason pelvic infections, infections of the womb, and rekindling of any previous pelvic infections can occur. Sometimes the infection can be treated by antibiotics without removing the I.U.D., but about half the time it is necessary to remove the device to treat the infection effectively.

Also, increased vaginal discharge occurs in a significant number of I.U.D. users and the presence of the foreign body (string) in the vagina makes vaginitis slightly more common. Recent studies by the F.D.A. have found that patients with I.U.D.s who do become pregnant run a high risk of infected miscarriage around the third or fourth month, and a significant number of deaths from infection with blood poisoning have resulted. The worst offender in this situation was the Dalkon Shield, which has now fortunately been taken off the market. The manufacturer of this particularly irrational device had done a tremendous selling job to the medical profession, and before its ineffectiveness and dangers were realized, several million had been used. In any event, should you become pregnant when wearing an I.U.D. of any kind, its removal and termination of the pregnancy by abortion as early as possible is advised. As yet there is insufficient evidence to conclude that I.U.D.s cause malformation of babies, affect subsequent fertility, or cause cancer.

Despite the above objections, the I.U.D. is still one of the most popular birth control methods used in the United States today. Once inserted, the woman has no further responsibility in her contraceptive program. It can be left in place for years if no complications arise, but I find that sooner or later most users do have one form of trouble or another. Although a semipermanent guard against pregnancy, women who elect the I.U.D. should have regular medical checkups, a good plan for all women, I.U.D. or no I.U.D. If you're wearing an I.U.D., riding in a car, and smoking cigarettes, then you're really living dangerously!

DIAPHRAGMS

Although oral contraceptives and intrauterine devices are more popular, the diaphragm and jelly is still one of our most effective contraceptive methods. In effectiveness it rivals the intrauterine devices, but it has none of the objectionable complications of either the I.U.D. or the pill. There are very few women who because of anatomical abnormalities cannot be properly fitted for a diaphragm.

Actually the diaphragm is one of the oldest known methods of contraception. An Egyptian papyrus dating back to 1850 B.C. described the use of a gumlike substance to cover the cervix. The modern diaphragm was invented by Dr. William Mensinga of Fleruens, Germany in 1882. It has since been widely used in Europe and was introduced into the United States by Margaret Sanger in 1915. Thus, medical experience with this method is extensive.

The diaphragm must be fitted by a physician, for the sizes may vary from fifty to one hundred millimeters. Also, the woman must be properly instructed in its insertion, proper use of the jelly and how to check the correctness of the position of the diaphragm. Most failures of the diaphragm and jelly method are due to patient's error rather than the method itself. As the diaphragm is not a completely occlusive device like the condom, it must be used with a contraceptive jelly or cream. Actually the main purpose of the diaphragm is to hold the jelly in place surrounding the cervix so that the sperm cells are killed before they can enter the womb. One of the diaphragm failures I recall was due to the use of the diaphragm without any jelly. (The physician had not told the patient of this vitally necessary step.)

By far the most common cause of failure is putting the diaphragm in the bureau drawer instead of in the vagina. Another failure I saw was a patient who assured me she had used the diaphragm every time she had intercourse. She was asked to bring the diaphragm in for inspection and it was literally in shreds, with a hole as big as a silver dollar in it. She explained that when she was not using it, her dog played with it and had bitten the hole in it. She did not realize that this would impair the effectiveness of the diaphragm! Also, as sperm in general can live in the vagina six to eight hours (I have even seen viable sperm cells in vaginal secretions twenty-four hours after intercourse), it is necessary to leave the diaphragm in position for at least six to eight hours after coitus.

On the minus side, a few woman object to the manual manipulations of their genitalia required by diaphragm insertion, and have the feeling that this is an unaesthetic method of contraception. Actually a well-fitted and well-placed diaphragm is hardly detectable by either partner. For those who anticipate cunnilingus prior to intercourse, there is apprehension that the taste of the jelly may be a "turn-off," but as these products are nontoxic, no harm can result. To prevent excessive drainage of the gel, I merely recommend the washing of the external genitalia after the diaphragm is inserted. It is rather psychologically traumatic to have to insert the diaphragm after foreplay has created arousal!

For single women, toting this "do-it-yourself kit" around on dates is rather unappealing. On the other hand, present packaging is usually like a compact or vanity case and can be employed almost as readily as the condom. For those with steady boyfriends this is not so objectionable, but for the one-night-standers, it is somewhat more of a problem.

The diaphragm is relatively inexpensive, for with proper care one might last a woman ten or more years. Once a manufacturer's representative showed me a testamonial letter from a satisfied customer that stated that one diaphragm had been used in her family for three generations! After removal of the diaphragm it should be washed with soap and water and filled with water to check for leaks. Then it should be carefully dried and powdered with cornstarch. In general, I do not advise douching after removal of the diaphragm. The vagina cleans itself by gravity; all that is necessary is washing the external genitalia. Some contraceptive jellies, particularly those containing phenylmercuric acetate, may darken—even blacken—the diaphragm, but this is harmless. Most contraceptive jellies are also effective in both treatment and prophylaxis against many vaginal infections. If you're scared of the pill and I.U.D., take a look at the diaphragm. It may be just the thing for you!

VAGINAL SPERMICIDES

Although somewhat less effective than the above methods, vaginal spermicides in the form of creams, gels, suppositories, and foams offer a simple local means of contraception. These are used without the diaphragm, but when used conjointly with the condom have an extremely low rate of failure. In using this method the woman merely inserts the measured dosage of the spermicide into the vagina prior to each intercourse with the applicators provided for that purpose. These preparations kill the sperm on contact and cover the cervix to prevent sperm from entering the womb.

The vaginal spermicides have several advantages: they are inexpensive; they can be bought without a prescription or fitting or instructions by a doctor; there is nothing to remove after intercourse; and douches are not necessary or even desirable afterward. Actually, douching right after intercourse considerably reduces the effectiveness of this method. If you have a compulsion to douche after this method, wait at least six hours after intercourse. In addition to their contraceptive effects the spermicides provide lubrication to the vagina and are prophylactic against several vaginal infections.

CONDOMS

The condom is so generally presumed to be understood that many pamphlets and articles on contraception do not even mention it. Despite the recent refinements in contraceptive sophistication, the condom is still the most widely used method in the world. It's not exactly new, having been invented around 1564 by an Italian anatomist. The first condoms were made of sheep's intestines, but since the development of latex the original "skins" have lost favor, although still produced. In addition to its high degree of efficacy (rivaling the I.U.D. or diaphragm and jelly) as a contraceptive, the condom is the only method that also gives effective prophylaxis against many forms of V.D. For this reason alone its use should be encouraged, particularly in the young sexually liberated.

The condom first came into widespread use in the last part of the nineteenth century, when it was employed by the armed services as a prophylaxis against venereal disease. This gave the condom a stigma of vulgarity which continues to exist. Printed on the package of some brands and on dispensing machines is the statement: "For prevention of disease only." Perhaps pregnancy should therefore be considered a disease! Many states still have laws restricting the sale or display of contraceptives, and about five states limit the sale of condoms for prophylaxis only. To insure the quality of condom manufacture, the Food and Drug Administration now has rigid controls which guarantee them free from defects. Unfortunately these specifications require a wall thickness of .05 to .09 mm.—two or three times the thickness of Japanese brands. Unquestionably the thinner product causes less loss of sensitivity, hence the popularity of the Japanese products.

In 1949 the Japanese introduced condoms of all colors (I could never understand how this could be a "turn-on" for any woman); they also come in a variety of shapes such as the plain end, the reservoir (nipple) end, and a tremendous variety of shapes and forms. Most ludicrous of these are the so-called "French ticklers." Perhaps no commercial item in the history of sexual folklore has been so overrated and exaggerated than these! They come in a variety of designs from tiny hands, porcupine projections, and multibulbous protrusions to actual extensions of the penis length and diameter. Their sale is popular among male sexual neophytes who have heard from some unreliable source that a French tickler would really drive a woman wild. This is a complete myth! More are sold as jokes and gags than for serious sexual activity. Actually the upper vagina is relatively devoid of sensory nerves, and most women are not aware of any different sensation with this ridiculous device. However, I have seen injury in the form of minor abrasions in the vagina from them. Moreover, the comical shape of the tickler requires a thicker product and the tip, which is the usual location of the tomfoolery, is so distorted that the glans penis is robbed of its high degree of sensitivity. What a rip-off! In essence, the man who uses this sort of junk is denying his own pleasure while doing nothing for his mate.

Condom failures do occur, but most of these are preventable. Since the precoital secretion from Cowper's glands in the male does contain some sperm, the condom should not be used only as a terminal method. It must be used throughout intercourse. Then, too, some men remain coupled until the penis becomes flaccid after intercourse, and the condom and its contents come off in the vagina. And, of course, without sufficient lubrication, the vigorous friction of intercourse can cause rupture of the condom. The much-feared "pinhole" is probably more imaginary than real. It is permissible to use surgical lubricants such as K-Y jelly with condoms, but any grease- or oil-based lubricant such as Vaseline must be avoided since these tend to weaken the rubber.

If you are contemplating adultery, give the condom a close look. It could save some very embarrassing explanations about how you contracted V.D. The time worn statement, "I got it from a toilet seat," is no longer acceptable, even to the most naïve. Then, too, the condom gives the male a prominent role in the problem of contraception—a long-shirked duty and responsibility.

DOUCHES

This antiquated and ineffectual method of preventing pregnancy is still used in some unknowledgeable circles. This includes such preposterous precautions as the Coca-Cola douche so frequently advocated by high school dropouts and college freshmen to their prey as an inducement to "go all the way." To be sure, a woman who relies on this method is foolish. As soon as the ejaculation occurs, the merry sperm are on their way to perform their appointed duty—to fertilize the hopefully present egg. Not only does the mad race to the douche fail in its contraceptive effort, it interrupts the intimate conjugation of the postcoital repose—particularly important to most women, especially if they have also reached orgasm. This method is mentioned in the text only as a matter of inclusiveness. Those who champion and believe in it are either stupid, unknowledgeable, or perhaps sterile from some other causes!

RHYTHM (Safe Period)

This method does not imply the tempo of the sex act—such as *allegro*, *largo*, or *dolce sostenuto*—but rather is based on a timing of intercourse to avoid the event of ovulation, such that fertilization of the hopefully unpresent egg is unlikely. Probably this is our most ineffective method of birth control. Although completely preconceived in its execution, it is probably no more effective than having intercourse to the strains of the "Poet and Peasant Overture" rather than to the stimulating rhythm of Ravel's "Bolero."

For many years it has been generally taught and religiously believed that ovulation for a woman with a twenty-eight-day menstrual cycle occurred around the fourteenth day. However, recent studies show that ovulation occurs much sooner—perhaps even the eighth to tenth day following the onset of the period; therefore, in one with periods lasting eight or more days, the egg can be present even before the cessation of menstruation. Thus not even intercourse during menstruation can be considered safe. I have seen patients who have limited their coital activity to only one day after and one day before their periods become pregnant.

Ineffectual as it is, however, the "safe period" is better than nothing (slightly). For those who do insist on playing this form of roulette, the basal temperature chart can be most helpful; that is, if you don't object to taking your temperature rectally every morning. As progesterone (the hormone produced by the ovary after ovulation occurs) raises the body temperature, one can tell from the rise in the basal temperature that ovulation has already occurred and that pregnancy at that time (or at least a day or two after) is unlikely. Of course, changes in the basal temperature can result from colds, flu, virus, or other infections; therefore, one must take these factors into consideration in interpreting the basal temperature chart.

Although the basal temperature chart is rather ineffective in predicting the fertile period for those persons who want to become pregnant, it can be an asset to those who wish to avoid pregnancy. It can be used only to establish *that* ovulation has occurred, not when! For those women who wish to use this adjunct to the rhythm system let me offer some suggestions:

(1) Buy a basal temperature thermometer. It is much easier to read because it is graduated in tenths of a degree rather than two tenths of a degree as is the usual clinical thermometer. Moreover, use the rectal thermometer, as rectal temperatures are more accurate and significant.

(2) Keep the thermometer on your bedside table and make sure that you shake it down well.

(3) Take the temperature rectally for five minutes before getting out of bed, talking, eating, drinking, or smoking.

(4) Take the temperature at about the same time every morning.

(5) Read the thermometer to the closest one-tenth of a degree and record it accurately on the chart.

The results for a normal woman with regular menstruation may give a chart such as shown in Figure I. Notice that the temperatures average almost a degree lower in the first half of the cycle than in the last half after ovulation has occurred. If ovulation does not occur, the chart does not show this biphasic pattern. As indicated, the fertile period is longer than generally taught and experience validates this concept.

Another usefulness of the basal temperature chart is that it is one of our earliest methods of diagnosing pregnancy. As is shown in Figure II, when sixteen or more days after the midcyclic rise in temperature the chart continues to rise, then pregnancy is probable.

Incidentally, the menstrual cycle begins on the day of the onset of the period, not when the period ends! Many women still count the days from the cessation of their menses to the onset of the next period as the interval between periods. It is not unusual for me to encounter a woman complaining of having periods every three weeks. When we find that her periods last seven days and begin every four weeks, it is clear that she does not have a problem of too frequent menstruation. Such mathematical ineptitude can play havoc with those people who are relying on the rhythm system.

Despite its sometime inaccuracy the safe period is without cost (other than the obstetrical care and rearing of a child in case of failure) and requires no special equipment or paraphernalia. It requires no physical examination, fittings, or financial incumbencies; and no ill effects, such as occur with some of the other contraceptive methods, can result.

For the woman with perfectly predictable menstrual periods this method can be used with a modicum of assurance if she avoids intercourse from the seventh through the sixteenth day of her cycle (starting with the onset of menses), but she would be more secure if she waited until the basal temperature chart showed about one degree elevation for at least two days.

To be sure, this is a regimented and premeditated act of pregnancy avoidance, but it is the only method of birth control accepted by the Catholic church. If sin is as the Good Book says,

FIGURE I

BASAL TEMPERATURE RECORD

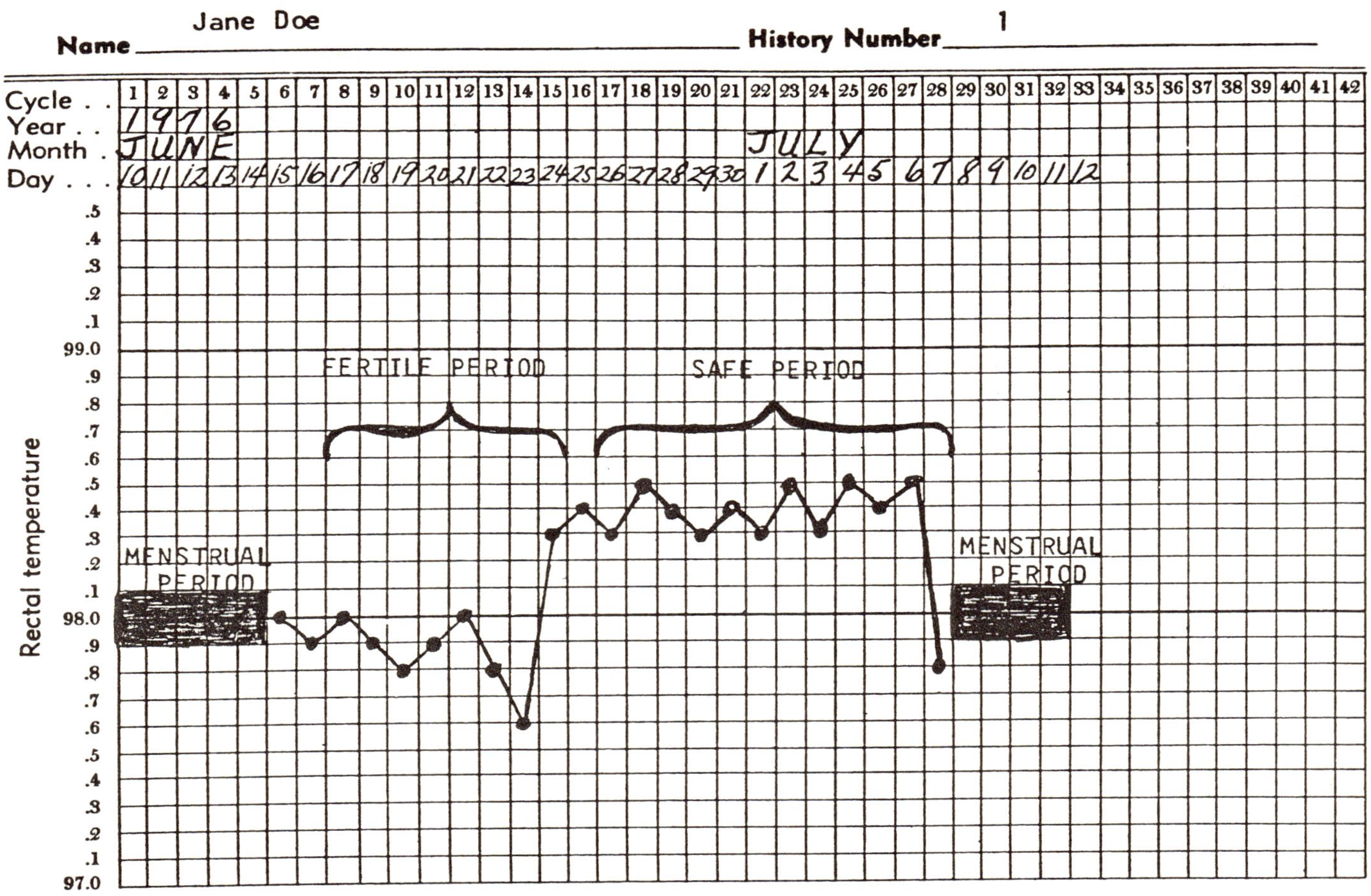

FIGURE II

BASAL TEMPERATURE RECORD
OF PREGNANT WOMAN

Name Mary Smith **History Number** 2

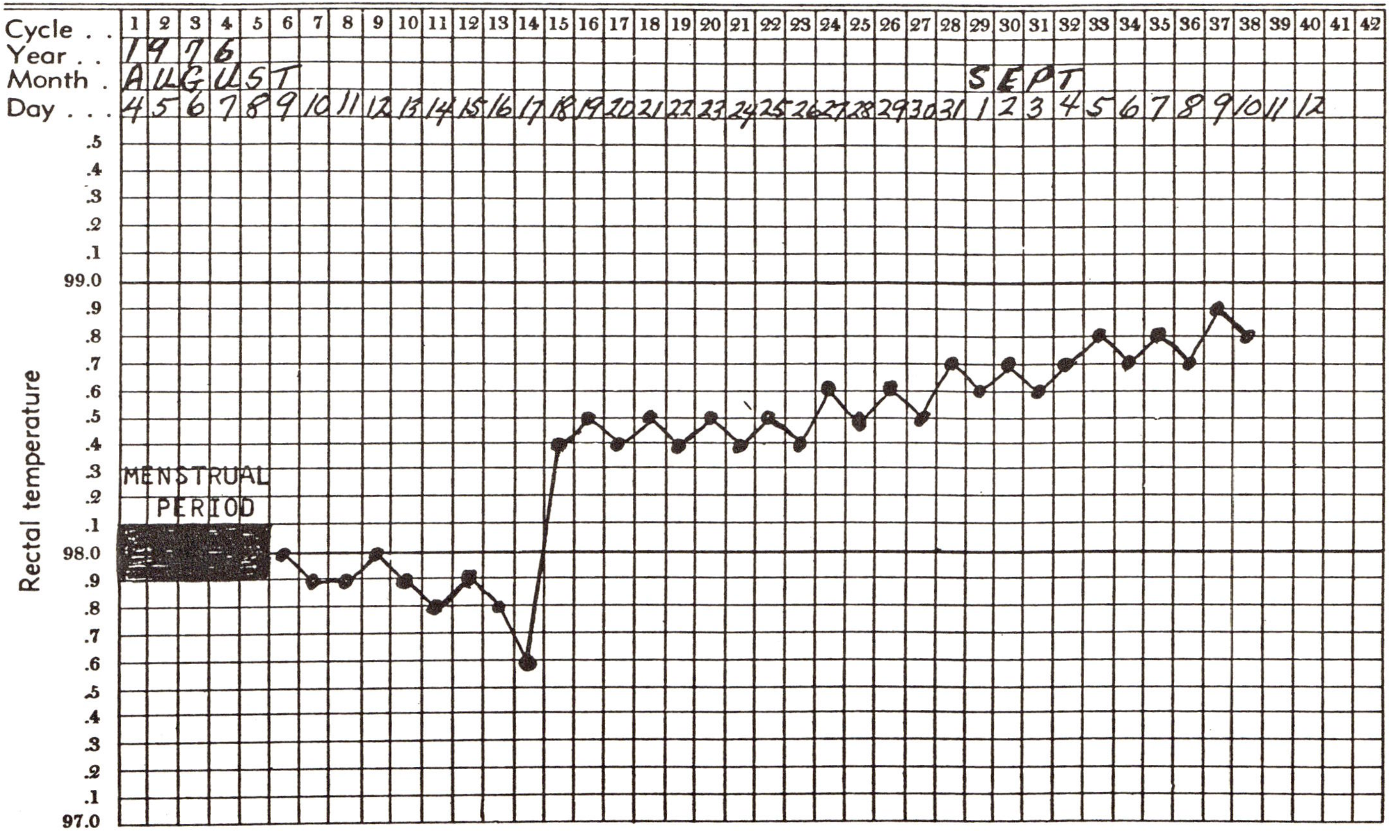

in "thought, word, and deed," then the only aspect this method avoids is the "deed." No doubt this is overshadowed by the increased proliferation of thought and word which would tend to vitiate the virtue of the "undeed."

In summary, I can say of the safe period that I have seen in my practice innumerable patients overcome with unhappiness because of the pregnant state resulting from belief in this unreliable method of contraception.

WITHDRAWAL (Coitus Interruptus, Pulling Out)

This is an ancient, somewhat effective method of preventing pregnancy, but its disadvantages far outweigh its advantages. Interestingly enough, in my professional experience this method is most commonly used by uneducated people who are frequently suspicious of, or disbelievers, in other methods. Commonly they are of rural backgrounds, and their sexual knowledge is so scant that they don't even believe women have or can have orgasms. With this method, they usually don't!

So important to a woman is the prolongation of the postcoital connection, which is, of course, impossible with withdrawal. I have seldom seen a woman to whom this method of contraception was satisfactory, and the very few who did had never known any other way! Besides its sad deficiency in being sexually fulfilling to women, its efficacy in preventing pregnancy leaves much to be desired. The pre-ejaculatory secretion from the penis contains some viable sperm and can cause fertilization. Furthermore, it is very difficult for a man in the throes of passion to be in sufficient control of his faculties to pull out in time. In any female-dominant position of coition this method is even more difficult to execute. It is not uncommon to see pregnancies result from coitus interruptus. If you're single (or even married and don't want to become pregnant), I would suggest some other method of contraception, both for its basic purpose, but more particularly so completion of intercourse can be carried to its normal conclusion and aftermath. Also, though I hate to admit it, many men, especially the single studs, can hardly be relied upon to use this method. Your best bet for safety is this: if he tells you he's going to pull it out, tell him he's not going to put it in!

SURGICAL STERILIZATION

Unquestionably the simplest operation for a family to prevent pregnancy is vasectomy, a simple office procedure that renders the man sterile—but not impotent. This operation is almost foolproof if the man is carefully checked afterwards to be sure that he is free of sperm. Actually, the ejaculate of a man is made up of only about 5 percent sperm cells, so the volume of the ejaculate is not significantly reduced. It actually varies a good bit from man to man, and even from time to time in the same man. Also the consistency, smell, and even taste are not altered by this operation. Unfortunately many men will not even consider this operation because of their stupid superstitions that it will render them unvirile, weak, and sexless. Nothing could be further from the truth. Of the doctors' families I know who have had surgical sterilizations, most of them have been by vasectomy. I highly recommend this procedure for stable, well-adjusted couples who have completed their families. On the other hand, for women who tend to stray, this method will surely fail; and, as a matter of fact, all of the vasectomy "failures" I have seen have been due to errant wives.

A frequent story I hear from women when I discuss surgical sterilization with them is that if something should happen to them, they wouldn't want their husbands to be sterile lest they should remarry and want to have more children. This is a rather martyristic and foolish form of logic. It's really tit for tat. Few women are looking for a husband with a whole slew of younguns, and those who are, seldom want to add more of their own.

TUBAL LIGATION

There are many different surgical procedures designed for rendering women infertile. Tubal ligation, which is one of the most popular operations, has many different techniques. The old wives' tale prevalent for many decades, that if the tubes are cut and tied, they will be safe, but if the tubes are only tied, failure is likely to occur, is hogwash! It is true that certain surgical techniques are more effective than others, but all forms of tubal ligation can and do (fortunately, infrequently) fail. Sometimes the operation is done through the vagina, but usually it is done through a small, abdominal incision. It can be performed at any time but is frequently done a day or two after childbirth. For the last few years tubal sterilization operations by laparoscopy have become very popular. This so-called "band-aid" operation is performed through a very tiny incision just below the navel through which a small, lighted instrument is inserted and the tubes are fulgurated (burnt), or a small metal clip is attached to them. This operation is simple and takes only a few minutes to perform; but as with all sterilization procedures in women, it is a major operation and complications can occur.

Since many women who have had sterilization operations do have later difficulties with menstruation, tumors of the womb, and even cancer, many gynecologists now feel that if a woman wants a sterilizing operation, this can be best accomplished by hysterectomy (removal of the womb). This can be done abdominally but is usually done through the vagina, thus leaving no scar. At the same time, vaginal relaxation due to childbirth can be corrected. It should be made perfectly clear that removal of the womb has no effect (other than psychological) on the sex life of the woman. The only effects of hysterectomy are inability to become pregnant and no further menstruation, which to most women is a blessing! Contrary to popular belief, the womb secretes no hormone, does not rid the body of any poisons in its menstrual function, and does not have anything at all to do with sexual or orgasmic function. It is also impossible for a man to tell any difference in intercourse with a woman, with or without a womb.

All surgical sterilizations should be considered permanent. Reversal of the procedure is difficult and usually fails (about 80 percent of the time) to accomplish the desired return of fertility. For this reason one should use the utmost caution and long-term perspicacity in considering any of the above operations. Hardly a month goes by without some patient consulting me, wanting her tubes untied. All too frequently young people with unstable marriages have this operation, later to regret it. As a case in point, a patient's husband told her after her second child that if she did not have her tubes tied, he would leave her. She had her tubes tied, and two weeks later he left her. She developed peritonitis after the operation and had to go to surgery again for a drainage procedure. Several months later she was seriously interested in another man, but he told her that if she could not have children, he wouldn't marry her. So she had another operation to "untie" her tubes. As is usual, this did not work. Some months later, she consulted me wanting another attempt to untie her tubes. I asked her what had the man done to prove his fertility? Had he even had a sperm count? When she said no, I told her that after he had had a sperm count I would consider her case. Of course, I never saw her again! How obsequious can one be to the male chauvinist pig! Permanent sterilization should never be considered as a last resort to save a marriage by women who have any marital discord. Don't be gullible and dumb. It's *your* body that is being worked on, and unless you yourself are 100 percent sure you want this for *yourself*, don't do it. If there is even the most remote hypothetical situation you can imagine where you could wish to be fertile, don't have surgery!

Hopefully the above considerations will be helpful to you in deciding what method of contraception is best suited to your particular needs. As abortions, though legal, are physically painful, psychologically traumatic, and more hazardous than contraception, the advice from here is, if you're going to have intercourse, contraception is your best recourse!

One of the unhappiest patients I ever saw was a mother of four who was advised by a "friend" where she worked. This patient had been on the pill for several years, was having semi-annual checkups, and was having no ill effects from the pills. Her sex life was completely satisfactory, and she had no fear of unwanted pregnancy. The so-called "friend," a person whom I found to have only a grade-school education, told her, "I wouldn't take those pills if I were you." On the basis of this quasi-sage comment, the patient stopped her pills. A few months later (this was before abortions were legal) when I told this woman that she was pregnant, she left a trail of tears from my examining room to my office. I asked her what the "friend" had advised her to do, but no alternative suggestion had been offered. Free advice is worthless, or sometimes worth less than nothing. Most usually, free advice is offered by unknowledgeable and intrusive persons who have some obsessive motivation to impose their ignorance, prejudice, or bigotry on the gullible. One thing I learned in twenty-six years of formal education is that if you want to know something, go to an authority for information. Don't ask or believe the opinion of one who knows even less than you do about the subject. The blind leading the blind is a pathetic situation; the dumb leading the dumb, even more so.

Although most women today are trying to avoid pregnancy, we still see many who wish to fulfill the greatest emotional experience a woman can have—motherhood. Sometimes it seems that the Almighty is unfair in that those women who don't want to get pregnant do, and those who want to can't! So fervent are they in their efforts that I even had a patient tell me that if I thought it would help, she would have intercourse at high noon on Main Street. Although I assured her I didn't think it could possibly help (and this was twenty-six years ago), experience over the years has made me doubt even this advice, for the psychological factors in infertility still defy specification.

It is well known and clearly established that the three basic necessities for fertility are an egg, a sperm, and a passageway for them to unite. Beyond these premises we fall into the area of conjecture. Although under normal circumstances the woman produces only one egg (ovum) each month (usually alternating from one ovary to the other), occasionally one encounters a woman who may produce two or even more eggs, and this is the cause of twins, triplets, or more. The new so-called fertility drug (Chlomiphene) causes a showering of eggs such that the incidence of multiple births has been far beyond the expected incidence. Although many people want to have *a* child, few people want to have triplets, quadruplets, or more.

Unfortunately, Chlomiphene is prescribed indiscriminately by some practitioners of general medicine (rarely by obstetricians) who have made no tests or even careful examinations as to the cause of the problem. This circumstance is aided and abetted by the insistence of women who have read in *Reader's Digest*, or some other pseudo-authoritative medical source, of the miraculous advantages of such a drug and insist upon taking it despite their lack of knowledge that the only cases it can really help are those patients who produce no eggs at all.

Nevertheless, infertility can be a devastating thing for a woman to admit. Sometimes it is even more so for a man, for his male-macho is at stake, but the facts show that of childless couples about one-half are due to male factors. It is very difficult to persuade men of the necessity for a semenalysis (sperm count). In the study of infertility this is one of the first and easiest tests that is performed. All men think that if they can ejaculate they are fertile, and to tell them otherwise, as is not too uncommonly necessary, is like a sentence of doom. Sometimes they even refuse to submit to the postcoital test of Huhner, in which the woman comes to the doctor's office an hour or more after intercourse for examination of the vaginal secretions for sperm, for fear they will flunk the test. In the management of numerous cases of infertility over the years, I would tend to agree with a large metropolitan clinic which found that the cases they had seen and not treated had as high a rate of conception as the ones they had treated.

Now back to the psychological aspects of the problem of infertility. Many years ago I was consulted by a patient who had tried to conceive for ten years. Her medical history revealed that she had experienced a criminal abortion as a college student, but since her marriage she had been very anxious to have a child. Furthermore, she told me that she had consulted a number of OB-GYN men before me and had already had innumerable tests, all of which had been normal. As she had undergone a recent examination I did not even examine her, but I did counsel with her for almost an hour about psychological possibilities as the cause of her problem. As an intelligent woman she clearly understood my advice. Three months later she returned to my office pregnant.

Once again I saw a patient that had been treated by a specialist in a large city who had performed even more tests than I was capable of performing. However, he prescribed nothing for her. When she asked if I could help her, my only thought was to prescribe a placebo (an inert medication that does nothing physically). Within a short time she was pregnant and has been so once since (on the same medication).

Although the primary prerequisites for fertility as stated above—egg, sperm, and a passageway—are basic, I have even seen impossible exceptions to these rules. For instance, a patient on whom I performed two hysterosalpingograms (X rays with dye injected into the womb) that showed no opening at all into the Fallopian tubes became pregnant.

Perhaps the best lesson I ever learned about the mystery, magic, uncertainty, and unpredictability of pregnancy was when

I was in Korea. One dismal Saturday night an infantry captain with a pistol showed up at my Quonset hut looking for my roommate, Dr. Jones. I told him that Dr. Jones was out for the evening and asked if I could help him. Why did he want to see Dr. Jones? "I'm going to kill him," the captain said. "Why?" I asked. "Well," he said, "he told Lt. Mary Smith that she couldn't get pregnant and she is." Never since then have I ever told a woman, regardless of her age, that she could never get pregnant.

I asked a mother of three, well-spaced children what she used for birth control. Her answer was that she had perfect conceptional control—a fact obvious from the spacing of her offspring. She said that she never conceived except when she had intercourse "doggie fashion" and that she only used this position when she wanted to become pregnant.

Even once pregnancy is accomplished, the desired outcome is not always attained, for about one in ten human conceptions ends in miscarriage (spontaneous abortion). Patients always ask what they did that caused this to occur, usually with a feeling of self-blame. This idea is abetted by admonitions from friends, even husbands, who know virtually nothing of the causation of miscarriage. If any form of exercise, diet, or drug would produce this effect, the million-odd women unhappily pregnant each year would have a simple solution to their plight. The most learned obstetrician-gynecologists have to use surgical means to terminate a pregnancy in its early stages.

Although there are some hormonal imbalances and general systemic diseases in women that can cause abortion, the examination of aborted fetuses in the pathological laboratory reveals that about three-fourths of them are abnormal—that is, not properly developing. A miscarriage is nature's way of arresting the development of an abnormal fetus. While such occurrences are generally attributed to defective eggs, there is no question that defective sperm can also cause maldevelopment. Although spermatic factors in abortion are difficult to define, most all physicians of experience recognize their existence.

For instance, a woman who had been married previously and had two pregnancies—and two children—married a man who had also been married before. His first wife had three pregnancies—all ending in miscarriage. The present union had produced two pregnancies, both ending in miscarriage. Another patient that had experienced three miscarriages was able to have a full-term baby after her husband was treated to improve his sperm.

Then, too, there are cases that no one can really understand. I was consulted once by a pregnant patient who had been treated elsewhere. She had previously had eight pregnancies, all terminating in spontaneous abortions despite all sorts of hormonal and other treatments. Her first question to me was, "What are you going to give me to avoid another miscarriage?" When I replied, "Nothing," she was quite upset, but with my reassurance that nothing else she had done had worked, she agreed to continue under my care. The baby, which she carried with no difficulty, weighed eight pounds!

The mystery of life and its beginning still amazes us all, particularly those who presumably know the most about it. For those who merely want to get on with it, the best advice I can offer is that if at first you don't succeed, try, try again!

CHAPTER 10

Surgical Selections

RECENT newspaper publicity implies that more than 2,500,000 unnecessary operations are performed each year in the United States at a cost of over $4,000,000,000 and a death toll of almost 12,000. These estimates are not based on medical audit figures, but rather by the mathematical techniques known as extrapolation whereby a small, and in this instance, untested, sample is multiplied by a nationwide figure to give a highly questionable answer. The presented figures in this particular situation were based on only 1,356 cases where two surgeons rendered opinions and there was almost 20 percent disagreement. (The very fact that there was disagreement between the surgeons does not necessarily mean the operation was unnecessary. At least one of them could have been wrong, but even this fact would cut the unnecessary figure in half!) Leading surgeons throughout the country have pointed out the fallacy of these figures; yet our Congressional subcommittee continues. In the words of Dr. Francis Moore, professor of surgery at Harvard Medical College, "They make two fallacious equations. They equate disagreement with surgical indications with lack of necessity . . . that's wrong. And they equate doing an operation on which there is disagreement with incompetence."

Actually, there can be frequent differences of opinions by doctors without either necessarily being wrong. As there are many ways to skin a cat, in addition to the hard-line, medical facts, the interpretation of these facts and projecting therefrom a line of treatment is influenced by the training (which varies somewhat in different areas of the country), experience, philosophy, and even the religion of the physician.

Of these so-called unnecessary operations, about one-third were hysterectomies. Of course, the crux of the matter is in the definition of the word *necessary!* There is no question that many women are having this operation for reasons other than to preserve life or limb, but on the other hand, there can be untold advantages to this procedure which our sartorially and oratorially resplendent solons refuse to consider.

It is beyond the conception of human perspicacity to equate so many units of happiness against the hazard of death. It is commonplace in our "now" society to covet living dangerously. Daring experiences such as skydiving are challenging. Every time we take a plane (or more hazardous, even a car), cross a street, or even breathe our impure air, we take a chance. Perhaps the destination, if worthy, deserves the risk. On the other hand, to be nowhere, to go nowhere, to do nothing or aspire to nothingness, imparts safety and consolation, but forever deprives us of fantasy, fun, and lifelong fulfillment.

To truly evaluate the table value of hysterectomy, women must take into consideration not only the immediate, surgical risk of the operation, but its lasting benefits. For instance, for the woman who has completed her childbearing career and suffers severe pain with menstruation and flooding with her periods, hysterectomy offers permanent release from suffering. Although

Congressional committees would probably categorize this operation as an unnecessary one, its benefits are unquestionably indisputable. To be able to enjoy sex thirty days a month rather than twenty-five, to be relieved of the tension, the pain, and at times the excessive demonstration of menstruation is surely a plus factor for this operation, not to mention its complete relief from the fear of pregnancy.

True, in many instances hysterectomy may be classified as unnecessary, but one can state categorically that *all* plastic surgical procedures on the breasts, *all* face-lifting or altering operations, and many orthopedic operations to alter or otherwise improve skeletal function are unnecessary. What then do we mean by "unnecessary" surgery?

Many times I have seen "necessary" surgery in order to cure cancer or some other fatal disease so mutilating physically or psychologically to the point that I would personally classify it a failure although the patient attained the medical status of "living and well."

The commonplace medical statistical tabulations of therapeutic results consider, unfortunately, only the survival aspects of treatment. The word "well" is a meaningless term. Perhaps a designation of return to a normal, happy life would be more significant.

As a case in point, I remember many years ago when I was an intern, we treated a woman in her early thirties for cancer of the cervix (neck of the womb) with radium. A few months later she developed a rectovaginal fistula from radiation burns (a hole between the rectum and vagina), resulting in constant seepage of feces into the vagina. The treatment of this condition required a colostomy (an opening of the bowel into the lower abdominal wall). After this she had to have another operation for the closure of the fistula, then another operation for the closure of the colostomy. Actually she was in the hospital almost continually for five years without a moment of pleasure, yet the statistical data presented by the cancer clinic listed her as "living and well" after five years of treatment. Is this really a therapeutic triumph or a tragedy? She never spent a really pleasurable day after her original treatment. Although statistically she was listed as a "cure," I would personally call her a failure of treatment. Yet all of her surgery was "necessary."

Many times in the surgical treatment of cancer we cure the disease but not the patient. Even though we render the patient free of the scourge of cancer but leave her nonfunctional as a human being, perhaps then our accomplishment deserves no praise. On the other hand, these operations are accepted as necessary to preserve human life and are unquestioned by Congressional committees (such as the House Subcommittee on Oversight and Investigations of the Interstate and Foreign Commerce Committee), the Department of Health, Education and Welfare, or jurors in malpractice injunctions. On the other side of the slate are operations performed to enhance the beauty, the self-esteem, and sensuous attributes of women. These are usually successful, the mortality minimum, and the cost usually less than a mink stole which alters only the exterior!

As one guilty of performing "unnecessary" surgery, let me cite a representative case. About twelve years ago I was confronted by a patient I had known for several years. As a matter of fact, I had delivered her two children. Her problem was an obsessive fear of pregnancy to the point that her sexual drive was nil. Various methods of contraception she had tried were unsatisfactory and also unreassuring. In addition she was having considerable menstrual difficulties. She stated that her marriage was in jeopardy and that I must help her. With her problem to heart, I suggested a vaginal hysterectomy and also asked if she would like to have her vagina tightened, as there was some relaxation from childbirth. Her affirmative reply justified to me the judiciousness of this "unnecessary" operation. I have seen her many times since, and a Christmas never passes that I do not receive from her a card of thanks and a reminder of the joy and happiness she has experienced since her "unnecessary" operation.

A trip to Jamaica can be dangerous, or Hawaii, or even New York, but it's fun. Sometimes a trip to the operating room can be hazardous but may result in fun, ego-elevation, self-esteem, and arriving. Only you and your personal physician can make the choice! Do not be bewildered by the sometimes unknowledgeable and prejudiced press.

Although unnecessary elective surgery can be a cause of death, it is also possible for it to save lives. The unnecessary operation for sterilization may have a risk to the patient, but may spare her a greater risk from the hazards of pregnancy.

From time to time many women—if not most—when confronted with the decision of having a hysterectomy (or other elective, gynecological operations) decide the best recourse is to obtain another opinion. There are innumerable gynecologists who would not stake their professional reputation for the sake of a single surgical fee. But most of all, the woman should expect—even demand—a clear explanation of the extent of the operation, the physiologic, psychologic, and sexual significance of the operation, and the specific and general surgical risks involved.

Next in frequency to the superstitions about pregnancy are the multiple myths and malicious misinformation disseminated to those who are contemplating or have had a hysterectomy. Foremost among these is the effect this operation has upon one's sex life. "You'll never be any good for your husband again," or "You'll never be a real woman again," are the common expressions in this part of the country. These admonitions are most frequently offered (and believed) by people of low educational and intelligence levels; however, it is surprising how many people of reasonable intelligence and high school or even college backgrounds believe such rot. With the multiple sources of factual information available today, it is hard to believe that people still believe in such foolishness. No doubt some women do profess a loss of interest in sex after a hysterectomy but they are only using this as a crutch—an excuse to justify their wanting to be that way—whether it be conscious or subconscious. Perhaps there is no more appropriate description of what actually happens than the age-old surgical retort: "I took out the baby carriage but left the playpen." The same evasion presents itself in the woman who gains weight after this operation. The fact is that the womb has no effect whatsoever on the sex drive of women nor does it in any way affect their metabolism. Any alterations in these areas depend on the psychological attitudes of the individuals and their dietary and exercise habits. And of course, these trends are aided and abetted by "brainwashing," distorted admonitions of neighbors, "friends," and members of their bridge and book clubs.

Another common myth ascribed to the operation of hysterectomy is: "It will drive you crazy." This it cannot do, unless your mind is already on the verge of emotional collapse. Then the stress of the operation plus the additional stress imposed on the woman by the constant barrage of busybodies can be the straw that broke the camel's back. For the most part, depression or any other mental alteration for which hysterectomy is blamed was already present and is merely exaggerated after surgery.

The indications for hysterectomy may be absolute, advisable, or elective (meaning optional, to be done at one's convenience). It is the latter two categories that difference of opinion and controversy might occur, but the word "unnecessary" is hardly appropriate. Examples of absolute indications would include cancer, large fibroid tumors causing excessive bleeding and pain, and other abnormal bleeding and painful conditions such as endometriosis, which cannot be controlled by other means. Advisable indications would include prolapse (droppage) of the womb, smaller, less symptomatic fibroid tumors, minimal degrees of endometriosis or just plain menstrual pain and flooding which sometimes does not respond to any other treatment.

In the category of elective hysterectomy would fall women who have completed their childbearing careers and perhaps as a result thereof have some degree of prolapse, vaginal relaxation, with possibly also menstrual difficulties. In time the prolapse and relaxation will probably become worse, and the added advantage of a permanently sterilizing procedure, in addition to the relief from menstruation, makes this a very attractive operation. Could this fairly be called "unnecessary"?

Sometimes religious tenets influence the surgeon and the patient in the decision to perform the hysterectomy. As no form of birth control (other than rhythm) is authorized and no operation performed specifically for sterilization is permitted by the Catholic faith, hysterectomy may be a compatible compromise, even on otherwise questionable grounds. This may be ecclesiastically sound but hardly scientifically appropriate. To pass laws restricting this type of indication would impose additional suffering on a significant portion of our population by taking away from them the only escape from the proliferation dilemma.

A memorable example of this form of rationalization was a patient whose priest refused to sanction a tubal ligation with her fifth Caesarean section but did condone a later hysterectomy on the basis of scar tissue in the womb (a result of the five Caesarean sections). This entailed the additional risk to the patient of another major operation, but gave her the solace of religious approval.

It is still commonplace today for women to select doctors on the basis of their looks and personality. Few women realize that the ugly, unpersonable doctor might be the most competent. Government statistics with which I agree imply that operations performed by inadequately trained physicians are more hazardous than when performed by "certified specialists." What does this latter statement mean? In twenty-five years of medical practice I have had only *one* patient call my office and before making an appointment ask if I were certified by the American

Board of Obstetrics and Gynecology. It is truly unfortunate that lay people do not know or realize the assurance and importance of the specialty boards. When dealing with your own health, the first line of defense is the family doctor or internist (currently called the primary care physician). However, now in some areas gynecologists are also considered "primary care physicians" for women. Even so, when there are surgical problems, consultation with a well-qualified gynecologist is appropriate. There are many trained specialists, and every woman in the United States today can have competent gynecological care.

For those women who don't know the significance of medical attainment let me point out the real meaning of a certificate on one's wall which reads, "Certified by the American Board." In addition to the four years of medical education, one must have at least four years of specialty training, must submit to the most rigorous, written and oral examinations rendered by only physicians of professorial rank in this specialty, and have clinical work with follow-up reviews for two years or at least fifty cases. Believe me, this is no "snap" examination. At the present time there are at least twenty-two specialty boards in the United States and although attendance to one so certified does not assure a positive result, at least one has the reassurance of having had "competent" care.

It is never amiss or even resented by the physician to have someone evaluate his credentials. When you "bet your life," you should be the final arbiter!

CHAPTER 11

The Genuine Gynecologist

A RECENT letter to Ann Landers implied that the most important men in a woman's life are:

1. Gynecologist
2. Hairdresser
3. Butcher
4. Furrier and jeweler
5. Husband

As an occupant of the top rung of the ladder, perhaps I should make some retrospective observations. To be sure, the gynecologist is a beloved confidant, friend, and confessor to most women but occasionally a mutation to the order occurs that tries to impose his own idiosyncrasies, pet approaches, prejudices, and inhibitions on his patients. Most women consider gynecologists, on the whole, to be a homogeneous group of physicians who deal with all women and their problems in a standard, acceptable manner. Not so! Gynecologists, as other physicians, vary in their philosophic, religious, and moral convictions. Despite the generally held presumption that all doctors, particularly gynecologists, are knowledgeable experts and masters of all matters of sexual prowess and performance, the divorce rate among physicians, including gynecologists, is as high, if not higher, than the general population; and this is not because of financial impecuniousness. In the preparation of this book I talked to many of my colleagues in order to enlarge my knowledge in this area. The responses I received were almost unbelievable. For instance, at a rather erudite meeting about a year ago I asked a man of considerable experience if he felt that anal intercourse was harmful. He immediately replied, "Certainly." When I asked him why, he thought and thought, and after a few minutes said, "I don't know why, but I'm sure it is." My retort was that this was surely a significant observation for a supposedly learned man of science!

Later that night, as we sat at dinner with a group of gynecologists and their wives, one of them, who professed to be an authority in psychiatry as well as gynecology, said that there is nothing wrong with women today which would not be solved if they had a five-inch penis. Obviously his knowledge of psychology was based on the Freudian concept of penis envy—a theory long before refuted and ignored. However, even if we consider the hypothetical possibility of such an occurrence, then all women (with their five-inch penises) would feel even more inadequate—as every *man* with a five-inch penis does.

Further discourse with a fellow colleague about sexual counselling as a part of our obligation to society produced the comment, "There is too much emphasis on sex today; I never waste my time talking to patients about it." (He had seven children!) To be sure, it is not so financially rewarding as hysterectomies, but it does offer a much-needed service which can impart joy and happiness to many. Sometimes just a word of reassurance or a simple explanation is all that is necessary to relieve the anxieties that the patient presents.

All too frequently physicians try to impose their moral, religious, and even bigoted viewpoints upon their patients. As a case in point, I received a frantic phone call from a patient (who lived some fifty miles away), crying and very upset because of a visit to a doctor in her area. I told her to come right over and I would try to help her with the problem. When she arrived I learned that because she could not reach me—I was out of town for the weekend—she consulted a local doctor. Having been a patient of mine for many years she did not realize that patient-physician communication should be repressed. Her problem was a severe infection of the mouth and throat, so much so that she could not even swallow. In her straightforwardness she asked the doctor if it could in any way be related to oral sex—whereupon the doctor gave her a half-hour lecture on the evils of such activity, even threatening her with the risk of cancer! No wonder she was upset; and he didn't even offer her any treatment for her problem. It was necessary for me to give equal time (one half hour) to undo the psychologic trauma that had been imposed upon her by her visit to a bigoted, puritanical physician (whose wife was probably even more so).

It is fortunate that all gynecologists are not like this man. By and large most of them are very knowledgeable and understanding, and they can treat people's needs whether or not they conform to their own standards or mores.

Long ago I gave up judging people, but rather trying to understand their philosophy and perspectives and offering help, not hindrance, to their lives. The homosexual or lesbian with gonorrhea should be treated the same as the heterosexual with the same disease. They do not come to the doctor for change of their sexual orientation or treatment for a preference no longer recognized by the American Psychiatric Association as a disease. They merely want treatment of their physical condition and this should be made readily available without the disdain or disapproval so often conjoined with therapy.

Sometimes one encounters gynecologists who refuse to give birth control advice to the unmarried (the ones I feel need it most) and moralize with them as to the evil of their acts. On the other hand, some are "pill pushers," I.U.D. enthusiasts, or diaphragm demons.

Ten years or so ago even my most communicative patients would rarely, or never, bring up sexual matters or problems to me, but now the pendulum has swung far in the other direction. As a matter of fact, rather than looking upon this with awe as I once did, I find the modern, forthright approach of patients refreshing and understandable. Furthermore, the patients' leveling with me as to the nature of their problems has made it much easier for me to give them the thorough treatment and counsel they deserve. Sometimes it means sadness, sometimes joy, but at least we can face the issues at hand and come up with a plan. Occasionally I encounter situations that are more like fairy tales than facts. For instance, a young, single, college student consulted me about a soreness of the vagina. After thorough examination I could find no evidence of disease, but only a slight redness of the vagina. When I reported to her that I could find no disease, she asked if her problem could possibly be due to "balling too much." Being familiar with such nomenclature, I nonchalantly asked how often she was doing it. When she said, "Five or six times a day," I replied that this could possibly be the cause and suggested that perhaps she should curtail the frequency. Her reply was, "But doctor, I don't think my boyfriend would go for that."

A married patient presented herself to me with a vaginal infection which on examination was of the sexually transmitted variety. Her husband had been in the hospital for some time with a broken leg. Naïvely she asked if she could have gotten it from skinny-dipping in the river. I assured her that she could, depending upon with whom she was skinny-dipping.

All in all, I suppose I have learned more about people from practicing medicine than was ever taught in the medical school. As a matter of fact, I believe many of my professors would be shocked at the encounters I experience almost daily. Some time ago a young, single, beautiful lady asked if she could speak to me about a very personal matter. I reassured her that anything she wished to talk about would be all right. Then she divulged that the only way she could have orgasms was to incorporate clitoral stimulation into her coital contact. I immediately reassured her that this was perfectly normal and that a good percentage, probably even more than half, of women need such stimulation to climax. I further added that this should not really be a problem, for all she need do is tell her boyfriend to stimulate her clitoris during intercourse. Her reply really shook me when she said, "But doctor, that's very hard to do with someone you don't know very well." Although I'm not moralistic, my devilish temperament impelled me to ask why she was in bed with someone she didn't know very well. Then she explained that on Saturday nights she liked to go to parties and have a few drinks and after several drinks she didn't care much with whom she ended up in bed. But as a last admission she did say to me, "Doctor, to tell the truth, those one-night stands are bummers!"

Another young student consulted me about not having orgasms. She revealed that she had been shacking up with a professor for six months. Once again my devilish, but not derogatory, demeanor prompted me to say, "Well, if you don't enjoy it, why don't you give it up?" Her reply was wholesomely motivated when she said, "I don't want to give it up; I just want you to tell me how to enjoy it."

A somewhat recent experience was with a patient in her twenties who indulged in, and enjoyed, just about every imaginable sexual activity. She asked me about shaving her pubis. I warned her about the dangers of depilatories, but told her that if she wanted to do this (at her boyfriend's insistence) it would not be harmful. The next time I saw her she was as smooth as a baby, but several weeks later I noticed that the hair was growing out again. I inquired about her enthusiasm for this caper, which at first had been all go, but after a little experience she found that she had to reshave every few days and that on the average she cut herself three or four times each trip—so the cracker crumbled. Over the years I have had very few patients who maintained a shaved pubis, and usually they gave it up after the novelty (razor-rash, abrasions, cuts and infections) wore off.

Although it would seem that the young have monopolized the sexual arena, let me assure you it is not so. A fifty-five-year-old woman (whose husband had had a vasectomy) asked me to assure her that she could not become pregnant, which I did. Further inquiry into her history indicated that she had been married for thirty-five years, had never had intercourse before marriage, and had never had any sexual experience except with her husband. Although she was happily married, the woman's curiosity had reached such a state that she contemplated an encounter with a man who had made advances to her. Later she confessed to me that she had done it but it wasn't so great. Perhaps it was like a touch of cement to tie her thirty-five-year bond even tighter.

I have learned a lot from these auditory experiences and have flexed to yield with the tide. Ten or fifteen years ago my insight and understanding were still impaired by "propriety." But all in all, I cannot feel that the present trends are all for the bad. A recent exposé of turn-of-the-century mores indicated that premarital intercourse was just as common then as it is now, only not so open and aboveboard as it is today. At that time it was undercover and sneaky, like closet nippers who never offer a drink to even their closest friends.

Fortunately, nowadays most gynecologists feel as I do about the rights of women to share in their medical problems and the decisions pertaining thereto. They have also progressed beyond the concepts of macho-mechanics and sincerely have a feeling for the feminity they serve. Really the only way for one to get insight into a doctor's dogmas is to talk to other patients he has seen, or even to ask his secretary about the doctor's feelings in certain areas. Frequently this can avoid an unpleasant encounter.

Having known many hundreds of physicians in my specialty, there is no doubt that the right gynecologist is a woman's best friend, and he isn't that hard to find—try your yellow pages.

CHAPTER 12

Don't Be Chicken, Be a Chick

ABRAHAM LINCOLN once said that you can fool all of the people some of the time and you can fool some of the people all of the time, but let me say that to fool yourself any of the time is dumb. In other words, don't let your mind get screwed up over screwing.

For thousands of years oral and anal intercourse have been used by some people to avoid pregnancy, and I might say that these techniques are extremely effective in this regard. In Italy where the population is predominantly Catholic, these techniques are used extensively, and for young, single girls this is a method of retaining (technically) their virginity until marriage.

Physically these techniques are probably harmless, but there can be psychiatric consequences. For instance, I once had a patient who had practiced fellatio and experienced cunnilingus for five years before marriage. She had an obsessive feeling that she should remain a virgin until marriage. Fifteen years and three husbands later, she was still unable to experience orgasm by penile-vaginal intercourse. In those five years she had established an orgasmic conditioning to cunnilingus, which had since persisted. I have never felt that the technical existence of the hymen was very important, but there still exists a small percentage of men who feel that virginity is one of the most desirable features of a prospective bride. I would not say it is an objectionable feature, but statistical data suggest that those people who have had sexual relations before marriage have a lower rate of divorce than those who have not.

Although the real weird, far-out, perverted practices are rather infrequent, there are many sexual impairments that are quite frequent and can cause a completely incompatible relationship. Premature ejaculation and impotence are the most commonly encountered examples. Some degree of fetishism, transvestism, and sadomasochism are rather frequent. Unfortunately, these latter preferences do not usually reveal themselves during the first few sexual encounters and can cause considerable concern—even alarm a woman when she discovers these tendencies. Some women can accept these activities as merely normal variations of sexual fun and games, while others will always consider them gross deviations and abhorrently perverse. At least a trial period of cohabitation prior to marriage could avoid these pitfalls. Also there are many women who can be stimulated to orgasm by some men and not by others, and this is not all a psychological reaction in the woman. Some males are too ignorant of female sexuality and so inept in technique as to be failures in bed. Whether or not one chooses to directly explore the sensuous appetites of the prospective spouse, at least a frank, in depth, all-inclusive discussion of all phases of sexuality should take place. One should probe the other's feeling about fetishes, flagellation, transvestism, homosexuality, anal and oral sex. Discussion of masturbation—frequency, technique, and associated fantasies—would be most enlightening.

The old Victorian concept that one needs to know nothing

about sex and that everything comes naturally is completely false. Dr. Alex Comfort so aptly implied in the *Joy of Sex* that a woman is no more likely to go to bed for the first time with no previous sexual knowledge and be a perfect coital partner than she is apt to go into the kitchen for the first time and produce a gourmet meal. Sex, like cooking, must be learned. Recent experiments with monkeys revealed that when both male and female monkeys were isolated after birth from the tribe and from monkeys of the opposite sex until adulthood and later put together, they did not know what to do and it took a long time—even months or years—before coital activity occurred. On the other hand, monkeys that were brought up with the tribe and had seen others in sexual congress had no difficulty in emulating their performance.

Most humans now have acquired by the age of puberty some degree of sexual knowledge—from books, sex education in the school (which I laud), seeing animals or even humans indulging in coitus, or by talking to friends. So at least there is some background for their embarking on the sea of sensuous expression. Unfortunately, a good portion of conversation regarding sex by young people is really a dissemination of misinformation, a situation aided and abetted by the inadequate or purposely misleading answers to questions they pose to their parents—the ones who also told them about Santa Claus, ghosts, the boogie man, and witches. A rather pathetic case I recall was a woman who came to me after two years of marriage to find out why she had not become pregnant. Examination revealed an intact hymen that would hardly admit my little finger. I advised her that the first thing she should do would be to have intercourse. When she replied, "I thought I had," I was stunned into speechlessness. However, with proper treatment and counselling, within a few months she had solved her problem and she was with child, but I never could muster the courage to inquire just what it was she had been doing for those two years.

It is every woman's prerogative to decide when and with whom, and I might add how, she wishes to have a sexual encounter. Sex should not be used as an instrument of appreciation, celebration, subjugation, or ego augmentation. Furthermore, the married woman should not view sex as a form of duty—an obligation imposed by the marital vows. In some respects many married women are actually prostitutes, demanding certain favors or gifts for intercourse.

Over the years I have seen many such women who complain that their husbands are sex maniacs—that they want to have sex as many as three times a week. I assure these women that this is only average and further add that the sexual potential of women is far greater than any man. Even prostitutes who do this twenty to fifty times a day suffer no ill effects (other than the disease potential).

For the obviously obstinate adherents to the sex-as-a-duty school I inquire of them, "If your husband comes home hungry, do you feed him? If he is cold, do you warm him? If he is unhappy or distraught, do you console him? Then why should he be denied the need of love and affection even to the extent of intercourse?"

Sex, like so many other forms of entertainment, should be looked upon as fun, a very special, personal form of fun, and should be savored in the true spirit of its meaningfulness. Today there is too much dependence on drugs or drink to release one's inhibitions sufficiently for them to participate to their fullest fantasy in sexual enjoyment and fulfillment. Actually this person is doing only what she really wanted to do anyway but could not muster the courage without an artificial crutch or boost. Thus, if a woman has sufficient bravado to be herself in the arena of amour, then artificial mind-altering agents are unnecessary, even undesirable, for a certain numbness and diminution of sensation usually accompanies them.

There seems to have been a timeless quest for drugs that

would produce aphrodisia. The oversexed or egocentric male feels that he needs an artificial stimulant to turn a woman on. If he only knew that love, tenderness, and gentleness are the keys that open a woman's body, he could give up his sterile search for the pot of gold at the end of the rainbow.

For thousands of years, alcohol has been considered to be an aphrodisiac. Actually it is like many other mind-altering drugs; it causes loss of inhibition and restraint, but cannot otherwise be considered a stimulant to sexual activity. Perhaps no better evaluation of alcohol can be found than in *Macbeth* (Act II, Scene 3):

> MACDUFF: What three things does drink especially provoke?
> PORTER: Marry, sir, nose-painting, sleep and urine. Lechery, sir, it provokes and unprovokes; it provokes the desire, but it takes away the performance. . . .

Cantharides (Spanish fly) was widely used by the early Greeks and Romans and is still considered by the unknowledgeable to be an aphrodisiac. Actually it is only a urinary tract irritant and can be harmful or even fatal. The Marquis De Sade killed two women with an overdose of this drug!

Strychnine, yohimbine, and many other drugs have from time to time been alleged to have aphrodisiac action. Like cantharides, these can produce serious or even fatal reactions—but not aphrodisia. Legend still prevails that certain foods such as oysters, mushrooms, eggs, etc., increase one's sexual potential. Not so! Actually there is no substance known today that is a true aphrodisiac; however, some women do experience an increase in libido from the male hormone testosterone.

Many of the patients that doctors see with various complaints are covering up, usually subconsciously, some form of sexual frustration. Headaches, backaches, intestinal disturbances, insomnia, pelvic pain, weight problems, fatigue, depression, and nervous tension are among the more commonly encountered examples. Frequently the patient herself will have no insight into the cause of these symptoms. All too often the doctor does not take the time to delve into the sexual history of the patient sufficiently to elucidate the true nature of the problem. He merely offers medication for the treatment of the symptoms which cannot possibly remove the cause.

On the other hand, many people nowadays because of increased sexual education and awareness realize that they have a sexual problem. To accommodate this group, sex-therapy or marriage counseling clinics are springing up all over the country. The vast majority of these are staffed by inadequately trained people, usually not physicians or psychologists, and frequently more harm than good occurs. Leading authority Dr. William H. Masters says that fewer than one in seven hundred can be considered legitimate; the rest are charlatans and frauds. If you do feel a need for sexual counseling, ask your personal physician or your county medical society for referral to a legitimate therapist. Let me caution further that although they like to advise in this area, preachers, for the most part, are totally incompetent to treat sexual problems. As a matter of fact, I have probably treated more preachers' wives for sexual discord than any other vocational group. To those who want to play doctor let me quote Luke 4:23: "Physician, heal thyself."

Sometimes women are confronted with one of their greatest fears—rape. If one is approached forcibly against one's will to indulge in intercourse, rather than fighting back physically it is sometimes easier to repel such advances psychologically by casually mentioning that you have a problem of diarrhea because of worms or the doctor has just found that you have V.D.

CHAPTER 13

How to Lose Weight

HERE is my answer to your weight problem, if you have one:

1. Don't eat!
2. Don't eat! Don't drink!
3. Don't eat! Don't drink! But make merry!

This seeming oversimplication of a major problem to a vast number of American women (and men), virtually unknown in most other parts of the world, is in essence a total, complete, entire, and singularly explicit remedy for this problem. Actually, everything that tastes good is fattening and should be summarily avoided. It is always an interesting insight into human habits to observe people in cafeteria lines. Without any knowledge of food value, calories, or nutritional aspects, an overweight person instinctively selects those items of higher caloric value, and conversely a thin person selects items of lowest nutritional value.

The untold millions of dollars American women spend on nostrums, quack remedies, diet pills, and shots to help with this problem are a complete waste! The American Medical Association's *Drug Evaluation Manual* clearly points out the inadequacies of "diet pills," and recently the F.D.A. disapproved the use of human choreonicgonadotrophin hormone (HCG) shots to combat obesity. Actually many diet pills are a derivative of "speed," an artificial central nervous system stimulant which causes undue nervousness and an excessive degree of activity because of the stimulation and a *temporary* loss of appetite because of the elationary effects of the drug. The long-term results are addiction, habituation, or dependence on an artificial crutch which has the end point of emotional letdown, increased dosage in an effort to combat the letdown, and increased weight gain because of the eventual wearing off of the appetite inhibiting effects of such drugs.

As a matter of fact, in twenty-five years of medical practice, I have yet to see one patient who, after six months, does not weigh more than she did before she took the pills. Yet the request is stereotyped—"Doctor, if you will only give me something to help me get the weight off, I'll keep it off!" Fantastic! My only motivation, admittedly erroneous, in prescribing diet pills is to get certain patients out of my office, for if one doesn't prescribe something, they feel you are not interested in helping them. They are not interested in diets, counselling, or common sense; all they want are pills. I have been rebuked many times by patients who claim the diet pills I prescribed for them are not doing their job. When I remind them that I never said they were "worth a damn," they always say, "Well, Suzie Jones takes pills and she loses weight." My reply is always, "Find out what pills she is taking and I will get you that kind." It is pathetic that so many people believe that if they could only take the right kind of pill, it would completely reverse their proclivity for gluttony! This is like looking for the pot of gold at the end of the rainbow. Fad diets, crash diets, all sorts of diets which are featured in almost every woman's magazines are, for the most part, worthless and at times dangerous. A low-calorie well-balanced diet with vitamin supplements has to become a way of life for the serious dieter.

Unquestionably the greatest "rip-off" in our supermarkets is the diet food counter. After omitting the expensive ingredient, sugar, most canned diet fruits cost more than their more flavorful counterparts with a saving of very few calories. Vegetables without salt cost more than those with salt; yet the amount of salt in regular goods is minimal. Diet bread contains only about 10 percent fewer calories than good bread. Furthermore, many so-called diet foods ignore one of the most important dietary restrictions—cholesterol. Nevertheless, many obese persons buy these foods religiously and thereby falsely justify unto themselves that they are actually dieting. Yes, one can get fat or even fatter on diet foods alone.

Another popular misconception is that polyunsaturated fats, oils, or margarines contain few or no calories. Although these produce less cholesterol, they contain just as many calories as butter or lard.

Recently there has been instituted an operation for the incorrigibly obese wherein the upper intestine or stomach is connected to the lower intestine or bowel. After this procedure is performed, the ingested food passes directly to the bowel so that frequent bowel movements passing the undigested food occur. This results in severe degrees of vitamin and other nutritional deficiences and can be very hazardous. Actually about 5 to 10 percent of these patients die within a year after the operation—a very serious risk for such a capricious effort.

In case you are like the numerous people I have encountered who say they can't quit eating, then perhaps you could at least excel in your indiscretion by becoming a world champion. In this respect may I insert that the world's largest human weighed 1,069 pounds, truly a challenge to the compulsive eater. You need not worry about clothes—Omar the tentmaker can cover everything. If food is the only thing that counts to you, forget the other aspects of living; try to be happy with your plight, just get bigger and bigger clothes and don't be upset by the criticism and disdain of others.

There are also many who claim that they inherited their obesity (yet weighed only five pounds at birth) and those who have glandular trouble (usually the salivary glands); but as a matter of fact, it would have been even beyond the most ambitious dreams of the alchemists of medieval times (whose main goal was to convert lead into gold) to convert water and air into fat. Perhaps my simplicity in approaching this problem is repulsive to many readers, but an infallible test I use in my office to evaluate the avoirdupois is the scale. The answer is very simple —if you weigh too much, you eat too much!

Another anthropological anachronism is the concept of being "big-boned." This connotation so commonly used as a justification for obesity can perhaps in general be understood, or at least misconstrued, but as a matter of fact it is impossible for a radiologist or anatomist to examine a human skeleton and estimate the weight of the living possessor of that frame. (We just shot that concept all to hell, didn't we?)

Another aspect of obesity that is not sufficiently recognized is the effect of liquor. Alcohol contains seven calories per gram and an average drink will have 150 to 250 calories, depending on the mixer. Most everyone knows of the "beer belly" now common, even in teen-agers. If you're really serious about losing weight, alcohol is taboo. (Incidentally it is also a powerful stimulant to the appetite.)

Frequently overeating is a result of unfulfilled needs, sexual and other frustrations, or general insecurity, and to be sure, such a victim is satisfied only by food—lots of food. The nervous need for something to do with one's hands, the craving for something satisfying, the urge to be fulfilled can ofttimes by relieved by the simple mechanism of masturbation. What a saving—no more food costs at appallingly inflated prices, no more drug costs for worthless nostrums, and no more medical fees for disservice for the treatment of a disease that defies the skill of medical science.

As an additional aid in losing weight, exercise is most important because it's not only how many calories you take in but how many you burn up that figures in the final total, and if you burn up more than you take in, you're bound to lose. The second law of thermodynamics (which the human body obeys) states that energy is neither created or destroyed, only changed from one form into another. Even simple walking burns up four times the energy of a body at rest. Incidentally, along the line of exercise, intercourse averages expending about 300 calories (the equivalent of a pint of milk). Thus, seduction can aid reduction.

Programs designed as consciousness-raising encounter groups that are really group psychotherapy such as Weight Watchers or TOPS, have made good progress in the treatment of obesity, and I laud their efforts. Unless a woman can put weight control foremost in her life, to seek its attainment above any other goal, she is doomed to the lodge of the large. As Arlene Dahl so aptly states in her book, *Always Ask a Man*, every woman has the will to weigh what she wishes. I wish you well in the fight against obesity which (I know) can really be hell. The psychological lift brought forth by a sensibly carried out plan of weight reduction far outshadows the tribulations, turmoil, and tedious suffering necessary to accomplish the end results. It can be done, and *you* can be the one who wins the battle of the bulge!

CHAPTER 14

The Waterworks

ONE of the most common diseases in women is cystitis (infection of the bladder). Symptomatically this causes frequent, urgent, painful, and sometimes bloody urination. Its importunate occurrence soon after marriage is commonly called "honeymoon cystitis." About 95 percent of the cases in women are caused by the colon bacillus, a normal inhabitant of the bowel and the usual bacterial flora of the vulva. As the female urethra (the tube leading from the bladder to the outside) is quite short (less than two inches) the thrusting action of intercourse tends to milk bacteria from the external genitalia up into the bladder where the infection occurs. Thus the honeymooner, or any woman indulging in frequent intercourse, is apt to develop this condition. As running water does not breed mosquitoes, the frequent turnover of urine in the bladder will do much to avoid this uncomfortable affliction. First of all, drink plenty of water. Remember when you were in the first grade in school and the health nurse said to drink at least six glasses of water a day? Then you were just a little kid. Now you need more. Second, *always* urinate after intercourse. In this way any bacteria introduced into the bladder by sexual activity are washed out before they can set up infection. Third, do not see how long you can go without urinating. By so doing you are producing a stagnation of water which is conducive to infection.

The common admonition by gynecologists and urologists that wiping after defecation from front to back rather than the reverse is helpful in preventing this disease is unsubstantiated. Although this might perhaps reduce somewhat the number of colon bacilli on the vulva, the fact is that the colon bacillus is still the normal bacterial flora of the vulva, and its presence there is universal. Nevertheless, the front to back wiping would still have an aesthetic desirability though not bacteriologically. It has been my fortune to rarely encounter patients who were so careless about their personal hygiene as to present themselves in my office with the perianal and vulval areas smeared with feces —not a socioeconomic relationship, for I've seen this even in the country club set.

Unfortunately some urologists consider cystitis in women an indication for urethral dilations. In the presence of acute infection this can be very painful, and as long as the woman can empty her bladder, could not possibly be helpful. Actually the very symptomatology of the disease causes too frequent (and complete) emptying of the bladder. Sometimes periodic dilations are recommended ad infinitum, until the woman finds of her own experience that this is not to her benefit.

As the urethra is often an erogenous zone in women and as a matter of fact its instrumentation is one of the common forms of masturbation in women, some do receive a vicarious sexual stimulation from urethral dilations. This is particularly true when the procedure is performed by a female nurse, for in this manner certain repressed homosexual tendencies can be satisfied. Most all people are to some extent bisexual, and I do not wish to knock it, but this seems to be a hell of a way to exercise one's subconscious sensualities.

Frequent and excessive dilations in women can result in such a stretching of this part as to result in incontinence of urine (loss of control of the bladder), which can be embarrassing both socially and sexually. Sometimes surgical correction of the condition is necessary.

Before the advent of antibiotics, urinary tract infections were treated merely by forcing fluids in large quantities, five to eight quarts a day, and surprisingly enough this cured most of them. The intake of lots of liquids is still the best prophylaxis against this all-too-common affliction. Remember; water is good for the waterworks!

Another common bladder problem in women—especially those of middle age who have borne children—is incontinence (loss of control) of urine, most particularly when walking, laughing or straining. This latter type is called stress incontinence. The original insult occurs in the stretching of the vaginal and surrounding tissues during childbirth. Later, usually after the menopause, when the loss of muscle tone in this area is furthered by the lack of hormones, the loss of urinary control begins, usually insidiously at first but with increasing severity. Often there is associated cystocele (herniation of the bladder into the vagina). Topically applied estrogenic creams in the vagina, or estrogens by mouth or injection, are quite helpful in minor degrees of this problem. But of more importance are the perineal exercises that strengthen the sphincter (cut-off) muscle of the bladder. To do this exercise, just try to stop the stream of urine once it has started. This can be done several times during each voiding. Once you have mastered the ability to start and stop the stream at will, the incontinence is usually relieved. On the other hand, neglect of the early stages of this problem and wearing of girdles will result in a gradual worsening of the condition over the years to the point where surgical intervention will be necessary. The fact that there are multiple operative approaches to treat incontinence of urine in women in itself attests to the inadequacy of all of them, for if any one operation was 100 percent effective, no other procedure would be used. At best only about 80 percent of urinary incontinence in women can be cured with surgery.

If used after childbirth, perineal exercises will do much to prevent the vaginal relaxation and loss of muscle tone which is a precursor of cystoceles and urinary incontinence

CHAPTER 15

Pubococcygeal Prestidigitation

ALTHOUGH anatomy books give very little space to describing the pubococcygeus muscle, sex manuals are verbose in describing the miracles of this muscle, which passes from the back of the pubic bone to the tailbone (coccyx). Some of its fibers blend with the urethral and vaginal walls and surround the anus. From a more practical standpoint, this muscle is the sphincter (contractor) of the lower vagina.

As we go downward in the spinal cord, specialization of muscular function becomes more obscure. For instance, one does not have nearly the control of individual toe movements as one has of finger action. The muscles of the perineum come from the lowest nerves in the spinal cord and cannot be exercised except as a group. It would be impossible for one to contract the muscles on one side of the body or the other, or to move one set of the muscles of the perineum and not the other. All of these muscles have essentially the same nerve supply so they can act only together. The bulbocavernosus (contractor cunni or sphincter vaginae), the sphincter ani, the levator ani (the main support of the pelvic floor and vagina, rectum and pelvic visceral organs), the pubococcygeus, the sphincter urethrae (which has to do with control of bladder function) all work together, and the contraction of these muscles always occurs simultaneously. Thus, any or all efforts to strengthen these muscles will give tone to all of them. By proper exercises, all muscles of the human body can be developed, and in the case of the female pelvic floor muscles, an increased awareness, appreciation, and sensation during intercourse can be obtained.

As a result of childbirth, or sometimes just from stretching from intercourse, these muscles may become lax and unresponsive. This can cause a decreased sensation to both the woman and the man. For the most part, the sensate stimulation of intercourse is due to friction; when the vaginal opening is relaxed, there is decreased friction. In addition to the anatomical causes, decreased friction can result from excess vaginal secretion and sometimes from contraceptive jellies, creams, or foams. Furthermore, some positions of intercourse provide more penile stimulation than others, and this is something each couple must work out for themselves.

At the time of female orgasm, all of the pelvic floor muscles contract rhythmically and involuntarily. This effect in itself will usually bring the male to orgasm. However, it is not necessary for one to await the climactic event in order to use and appreciate the pelvic floor muscles. Simple exercises can be readily learned which can give more voluntary control and tone to this area.

In general, the contraction of the pelvic floor musculature occurs when one attempts to cut off the stream of urination or stop a bowel movement. One of the simplest and most effective methods of exercising these muscles is to urinate with the legs apart and to try to stop the stream several times in the course of voiding. (Do not feel inadequate if you fail the first few times. Few people can juggle five balls without practice.)

Another helpful exercise is to lie on the bed on your back, elevate your hips off the bed and contract the muscles as if to stop a bowel movement. As with all forms of exercise, persistence leads to perfection so don't be discouraged. Keep trying!

Although instruments have been devised to actually measure the strength of the pubococcygeal contractions, these are not necessary in order to accomplish the desired results. One can merely insert two fingers in the vagina and perceive the intensity of the grip—or even one finger, for that matter.

Particularly for those who have borne children where the vaginal muscular supports may have become overstretched, these exercises are a must, both to the sensual satisfaction of the male and the woman herself. At the time of female orgasm, the involuntary and even violent, rhythmic contraction of these muscles occurs and is a tremendous enhancement of this experience to both man and woman. A little preconditioning reflects the Boy Scout motto: "Be Prepared."

One should practice contracting these muscles for a count of three and also flicking them back and forth as rapidly as possible. In addition to the muscular control, the performance of these exercises focuses a woman's attention to an important part of her body and makes her more aware of the potential of this area.

Another exercise which I like to recommend is to stand erect with both hands on the buttocks. In this situation you can actually feel the elevation of the buttocks by the contraction of the muscles. When you have mastered the rapid flicking of these muscles, and when you can engage in intercourse to the total satisfaction of yourself and your lover without any other movement, then you have really mastered the magic of pubococcygeal prestidigitation.

CHAPTER 16

Masturbation Myths

MASTURBATION does *not* cause:

1. Insanity
2. Acne
3. Blindness
4. Hair growth on the hands
5. Nervous exhaustion
6. Retarded or stunted growth
7. Nymphomania
8. Death

On the other hand, masturbation *does* cause:

1. Sexual self-awareness
2. Opening of the orgasmic door
3. Relief of menstrual cramps
4. A substitute for overeating
5. Relief from nervous tension
6. Fun

Medical texts as late as the turn of the century described

masturbation as self-abuse, self-pollution, a pernicious and ruinous solitary vice. All sorts of afflictions were ascribed to it. Krafft-Ebing, in his *Psychopathia Sexualis*, a book devoted to the most bizarre and abnormal sexual crimes, errantly deduced that masturbation was the cause of those perversions, since most all of the sex criminals he examined had started to masturbate at an early age. It's too bad that he didn't have the Kinsey report, for then he would have known that most normal people also begin to masturbate at an early age. At the present time, most physicians would consider the young nonmasturbator the abnormal one. Even so, some parents still condemn children for this practice and threaten them with the evil consequences that can result therefrom. This imposes upon the child a distorted impression of her sexual organs and inflicts upon her the erroneous concepts that the sexual organs are untouchable and that everything associated with sex is dirty. What greater impetus to the development of an inferiority complex and low self-esteem could there be than to think of one's own birth as begotten by an act of filth?

In the nineteenth century numerous ingenious antimasturbation girdles were used for both males and females. Such items as the Buster Brown Anti-Pollution Panties, Mother Agnes's Chastity Girdle, and Mrs. Flanagan's Nightbelt for Maidens were some of the commercially available contrivances imposed on children by overprotective (and stupid) parents in order to "save" them from the evils of self-abuse. Krafft-Ebing reported a case to illustrate the obstinacy of this degenerate disease. He called it "the disgusting story" of a girl who began to masturbate at seven, and "at the age of ten was given to the most revolting vices. Even a white-hot iron applied to the clitoris had no effect in overcoming the practice." What more barbaric and sadistic action could be imagined? Today Krafft-Ebing himself would be considered a pervert, morbidly preoccupied with the sexually terrifying and disgusting. Yet he had a tremendous influence on the medical and social thinking of his time. Even today many parents still impose various punishments and remonstrations on children for performing this normal (and even beneficial) bodily function.

For those who are hard of hearing, let me reiterate; masturbation is normal! In addition to its pleasurable attributes, masturbation can frequently relieve menstrual cramps by detumescing and decongesting the womb and pelvic organs through orgasm. Furthermore, for those who are prone to overeat because of a nervously deprived condition and a desire to do something with their hands, masturbation offers an ideal, nonfattening outlet. Yes, masturbation is *normal!* Particularly for the feminine self-pleasurist, it enlightens her as to her anatomy, the erogenous responsive potential of her body, and imparts the otherwise aforementioned advantages. Unlike the male, women masturbate in a variety of ways. Manipulation of the clitoris or the surrounding area is the most common. Only a limited number of women employ phallic substitutes for this practice. Actually, a woman should vary her method of masturbation; the constant conditioning to one method might limit her sexual versatility and could impair the ultimate attainment of penile-vaginal orgasm.

Some women prefer direct clitoral stimulation, but others find the clitoris so sensitive that only the adjacent tissues produce the desired response. Xaviera Hollander says her favorite method of masturbation is to lie in the tub with her legs up and the stream of water directed on her clitoris. For those fortunate few who have a bidet, a most pleasurable sensation can be experienced. Whatever your preference, it's all normal and like all bodily functions you should "know thyself." Once you have an insight into your own sexuality it is very simple to communicate your needs to your partner. Show how you masturbate; tell what you would like. It should be no more of a put-down than telling someone how you want your steak cooked.

For the sexually unenlightened, may I affirm that *all* female orgasms are clitoral. The Freudian concept of the "mature" vaginal orgasm is a myth. Probably more than half the women require some clitoral stimulation during intercourse in order to attain orgasm. If you are one of these, you're not inferior. Just tell your mate what you need or do it yourself. It's still normal.

A question I am often asked is what is normal in regards to the frequency of masturbation. As with all other sexual outlets, the normal depends on one's individual needs. For some women, once every week or so is enough, while others may require ten or more times a day. Frequently women will experience multiple orgasms at each session before they are satisfied. There is no such thing as excessive masturbation *causing* neurosis; on the other hand, excessive masturbation can be a symptom or manifestation of neurotic disease.

Women, more than men, envision fantastic fantasies during the execution of masturbation. Daydreaming of knights in shiny armor on white steeds, gang rape, or even bondage subjugation are not uncommon forms of such hallucinations. Once again, this is normal—even desirable—for in this way one can express, even experience, one's true sexual identity. Furthermore the brain, the most important sexual organ in the body, is thereby utilized in the act.

VIBRATIONS

Not the sexually attractive, nondescript, adhesive magnetism that brings even sometimes strangers together, or the horrible horoscopic signs that are reputed to influence the sensuality of the mind, or the body chemistry which is supposed to repel or reject as the case may be, or the deafening drone of acid rock, but rather the mechanical dynamic scintillations produced by the gadgets called vibrators. As an adjunct to sexual play, these are truly fun things, but as many other tribulations of living they have both good and bad points. For the nonorgasmic woman (R.I.P.) sometimes they can open the door to a new world of sensuous delight. On the other hand, habituation to this artificial means of orgasmic fulfillment can impair one's relationship with the opposite (or even same) sex.

Although the motorized phallic symbol is the most frequently advertised (and thereby sold) type of vibrator, this is the lowest on the totem pole of approval for its effectiveness. Although battery-operated and portable, they are much less intense in their stimulating power than the corded gadgets that strap on to the hand or present a rubber disc for direct or indirect clitoral stimulation. The male myth that most women masturbate with phallic substitutes even permeates the manufacturing market of sexual aids.

Many sex therapists recommend the use of vibrators—particularly for the nonorgasmic female, as many women have learned to realize their orgasmic potential by means of these devices. The massagers which strap on to the hand also give the fingers a role in this endeavor. (But sometimes the hand can be numbed by the violence of the vibrations.)

The reactions of men to vibrators are variable. The more liberated males like to use any means available to impart to their consorts as much pleasure as possible. At the other end of the spectrum are those who have an intense jealousy and disdain that a mechanical gadget can give more stimulating response than they themselves. Thus a male antimachismo, impotence, or inferiority can occur. For this reason many women tend to conceal their vibrator vicissitudes. It's best to know your man before you try!

CHAPTER 17

Old Wives' Tales —Retold

ALMOST everyone, despite his intelligence, occasionally indulges in the fantasy of superstition. Even when one knows the fallacy of such beliefs, he conforms to them and passes them on to others, thus perpetuating the myths.

Although some signs such as finding a horseshoe or a four-leaf clover are supposed to bring good luck, most omens foreshadow bad luck. The meeting of a black cat, the breaking of a mirror, the opening of an umbrella indoors, or walking under a ladder are universally accepted examples. The widespread aversion to the number 13 is so ingrained in our society that many people avoid motel rooms, house numbers, phone numbers, and many other numerated things because they contain this number. Particularly prevalent is the fear of any Friday the thirteenth. Most of these silly superstitions are harmless, for the most part, and few people take them too seriously. On the other hand, when unfounded beliefs are presented that can cause one grief, undue fear, or even psychologic anxieties, then a great disservice has been done. Probably in no area is this form of inhuman imposition more abundant than in the many myths concerning pregnancy. Despite the popular prevalence of these notions, textbooks of obstetrics do not mention them and the medical literature is particularly devoid of references in this area.

More chastising than the hazing initiation into any sorority is the "brainwashing" introduction into the society of motherhood. It has long been perversely prevalent—perhaps even considered by some as proper—to plague the potential mother with innumerable misquotations, superstitions, and even prefabricated prevarications—generally classified as "old wives' tales."

To the young, unknowledgeable woman, pregnant for the first time, the contemplation of the very experience itself is sufficiently awe-inspiring. It is particularly inappropriate for older people (usually women and especially old maids—the world's leading authorities in obstetrics) to augment the natural apprehension with sadistic impositions of which most, if not all, are 100 percent phony.

Old wives' tales possibly originated with, but surely have been perpetuated by, untrained, uneducated midwives whose total contribution to humanity would probably balance out on the minus side. Usually their prevarications were fabricated in order to cover their own inadequacy, inexperience, and unknowledgeability. One of the most difficult statements for a professional (or pseudo-professional) person to make is, "I don't know." Generally unacceptable to lay people and as an admission of incompetence, it is a natural effort on the part of those with only *slightly* more knowledge than the other person to explain away any deficiency on their own part by passing the blame onto the unsuspecting innocence of the naïve. Until a few decades ago this practice was even indulged in by many physicians. (Sometimes I have wondered whether they really didn't know any better or were purposedly perjuring themselves!)

It has always been very easy to explain to the parent that

the fatal fetal outcome of a pregnancy was due to strangulation by the umbilical cord around the neck—a condition generally accepted beyond question even today as a certain unequivocal cause of death for the baby. Probably even the legend of Santa Claus has not had the widespread, worldwide publicity as the well-accepted, generally understood, unfactual presumption that if a pregnant woman reaches up over her head or bends over, this can cause the umbilical cord to wrap around the neck of the baby. Thus the blame for the unfortunate outcome is bestowed upon the mother. Already bereaved in her loss, she now has to endure the guilt of the causation of the disaster. The midwife or doctor is thus still exalted and exonerated.

The fact is that during pregnancy the baby has complete freedom of movement within its pool of amniotic fluid contained within the womb. It can turn somersaults, handsprings, twirls, and all sorts of gyrations imaginable. These are *not* related to the activities of the mother. Even if the mother is lying at rest, the activity of the fetus continues, completely beyond her control. During these activities it can well be appreciated that at times (statistically about one out of every three or four) the cord will be wrapped around the baby's neck. If the cord is long, the baby can pass through a loop in the cord, producing a knot.

Alarming as these *facts* may seem, they are rarely fatal. It is not uncommon for the obstetrician to encounter three or four loops of cord around the baby's neck without ill effect, and knots in the cord are fairly frequent. One cannot compress the arteries to his own head and cause death (because as soon as unconsciousness occurs, relaxation occurs), nor can the baby strangle itself. Still, it will probably be another century or two before the myth of the "cord around the neck" is completely squelched.

Since the beginning of time, much mystery has shrouded the miracle of birth and, unfortunately, the superstitions have surpassed the factual understanding in general dissemination. Even the learned physician Hippocrates, considered the father of medicine, wrote that if a woman is pregnant with a son, she has a better color, moves with more ease, and her right breast is bigger, firmer, fuller, and the nipple more swollen. However, if she is pregnant with a daughter, there is pallor and the left breast, particularly the nipple, is more enlarged.

Although today we can look back on these ridiculous presumptions as preposterous, we are still not completely enlightened. The shadow of the Dark Ages still enshrouds us. Incidentally, during the Dark Ages it was presumed that the human baby gained access to the outside world by its persistently increasing muscular activity resulting in its delivery, such as the baby chick eventually breaks out of the egg.

Another equally ridiculous "belief" concerning pregnancy is the concept that if a pregnant woman should look at fire or a corpse, the baby will be "marked." Actually there is no connection between the nervous system of the fetus and the mother; therefore no psychological experience of the mother can possibly be transmitted to the baby. Moreover, there is normally no interchange of blood between the mother and the fetus. Their circulations are completely independent of one another but nutritive interchange occurs through the membranous filaments of the placenta which are called villi. The natural craving of pregnant women for certain foods (pica) has at times been condemned as an avenue to disaster. It is common knowledge that if a woman has a craving for strawberries and does not get them, the baby will have a strawberry mark. It is even risky for the husband to fail to provide for whatever craving his wife desires lest he endure an endless barrage of accusations and chastisement by the busybodies, friends, and relatives. Perhaps the most ridiculous "belief" I have ever heard was about a pregnant woman who once ate a lobster, and the child was born resembling a lobster. I think I could believe in witchcraft quicker than that! Despite the admonitions of the busybodies, the *diet of a pregnant woman in no way affects the outcome of the pregnancy so far as the baby is concerned.* Actually, the fetus is a complete parasite and whether or not the mother gets adequate nutrition the baby will. During World War II the pregnant women in German concentration camps, fed on only bread and water, for the most part had healthy babies.

Many women still believe that the occurrence of birthmarks represents incidents in the mother's pregnancy. One can always reflect on the many, many things that the mother did, felt, or saw during the pregnancy, and invariably some tidbit of trivia can be revived which, to many unenlightened ones, would adequately explain the occurrence. If every incidence encountered in the nine months of pregnancy caused a mark on the baby, we would all look like leopards. There are also stories of deliberate attempts to "mark" babies, particularly in the medieval days of religious fervor when pregnant women burned crosses on their bodies in order to have "holy babies" so marked; however, none of these efforts were successful in producing the desired results.

The felicitations usually offered to pregnant women by friends, or more usually casual acquaintances, should really be considered affronts rather than greetings. A comment such as, "You're much too big for your time (or small)," is a common example. Never have I seen a pregnant woman who was assured by her peers that her size was just right! Another admonition by the pseudo-knower is, "You're carrying the baby too low (or too high, as the case may be)." As an obstetrician of a quarter century's experience I have yet to learn the significance of carrying a baby high (or low), although some people claim to be able to determine the sex of the child this way. I don't recall whether it is a boy or a girl that is carried high or low. As a matter of fact, in my extensive observation of pregnant women, I have never been able to even detect the high or low carriage either from casual observation or careful physical examination—a permission not generally extended to the pernickety personalities so gifted with presumptuous predictions.

Another common fallacy among women is that boy babies originate from the left ovary and girl babies from the right (or vice versa). Anyone with even part of his bag of marbles knows that women with only one ovary can—and do—have babies of both sexes.

For some reason it has been deeply instilled into lay thinking that a premature baby born at the seventh month is more likely to survive than one born at the eighth month. All medical, logical, and statistical data positively refute this ridiculous concept. On the other hand, it is not uncommon now to see many babies who weigh six, seven, even eight or more pounds born in the seventh month—*after marriage!* Perhaps these births have always occurred and have formed the basis for this erroneous belief.

Everyone knows—especially the astrologically oriented person—that more babies are born during the full moon—a myth even substantiated by delivery-room nurses and a few doctors. To be sure, because of the romantic inspiration of the full moon, more babies may be conceived at this time, but there is no evidence that there are more deliveries at this occurrence. Furthermore, the common misconception that more babies are born at night is statistically invalid. Once again, perhaps more babies are conceived at this time but not delivered. Since the duration of labor, particularly with the first baby, exceeds twelve hours, at least part of the lying-in is at night—a fact that perhaps interferes with the sleep of the obstetrician but in no way correlates with birth timing. As a matter of fact, the statistical data based on very large numbers of deliveries indicate that there is no consistent seasonal, lunar, or temporal distribution. Babies are born with equal frequency around the clock, the phases of the moon, the vernal equinox, solar eclipses, or whatever other fantastic figuration might be postulated. Regardless of the time of its occurrence, a knife under the pillow will not "cut" the pain of labor, nor will the age-old techniques of "snuffing" or "feathering" speed it up.

One aspect of obstetrics that has been perpetually fascinating is the prediction or the predetermination of the sex of the offspring. For almost a century it has been accepted that the fetal heart rate is a reliable method of predicting the sex of the baby. I believe the concept is that a fast beat in the order of 140 beats per minute indicates a girl, whereas a slower rate such as 120 beats per minute indicates a boy. This myth is still perpetuated by many delivery-room attendants and even some physicians. The fact is there is no difference in the fetal heart rate of male and female babies and rather than a sign of sex, alterations in the fetal heart rate may herald impending distress to the child!

Even more ethereal are the efforts to predetermine the sex of the baby. The acid or alkaline douches prior to intercourse probably have more effect in preventing pregnancy than in predetermining its outcome. The programming of intercourse for this purpose—so many days after the period for a girl or so many for a boy—is equally ineffectual; studies show no better than chance expectancy for these efforts.

Nevertheless, it is now possible with the technique of amniocentesis (a procedure wherein a needle is passed through the abdominal wall of the pregnant woman into the womb withdrawing some of the amniotic fluid) to not only determine the sex of the baby but also in many instances to tell if the baby is defective.

There is unquestionable evidence that certain drugs taken in the first three months of pregnancy can cause malformations of the baby and that undue exposure to X rays can also cause such results. Some infectious diseases, especially German measles, during the developmental stages can cause very serious malformations. On the other hand, most malformations of the human fetus are due to causes yet unknown. The fear of a malformed or mentally deficient child is surely one of the greatest apprehensions faced by every pregnant woman. Statistically speaking, however, malformations occur only about one in two hundred cases; in other words, your chances are 99.5 percent the baby will be normal. Even so, no pregnant woman should take any drug—even aspirin—without consulting her physician. Furthermore, one in anticipation of pregnancy should not have elective X-ray studies except during the first ten or twelve days after the onset of menstruation.

Besides the possible contributing causation of malformation by drugs and X rays are hereditary factors. Particularly is this true with regards to the extremities (arms, legs, toes, and hands). I once encountered a case where for three generations there were two fingers missing on the left hand. Surely this was a familial tendency.

One other factor in the development of a specific malformation, namely the Mongolian idiot, is the age of the expectant mother. It has been statistically shown that women pregnant for the first time at the age of thirty-five and over have an increasing hazard of this possibility, especially as their age advances.

Another common misconception about conception is that sexual intercourse during the first three months can cause abortion, particularly if indulged in at the time of expected menstruation. If only this were true, the 1,000,000 women in the United States unhappily pregnant each year could solve their problem by just having additional sexual activity. (*Don't count on it. It won't work!*)

Only after you have experienced a few pregnancies can you really know what it's like. No longer are you gullible about the stupid superstitions imposed upon you in your innocence. Hopefully you, as a happy mother, will not pass on to your juniors the horrendous horrors of "old wives' tales."

CHAPTER 18

Aphorisms on Momism

MODERN communications technology is truly remarkable. We can transmit verbal and pictorial images via telecommunication satellites almost instantly around the world and even to our astronauts on the moon. By the miracles of recording techniques we can still experience the dynamic artistry of Caruso or Lily Pons. Even the fireside chats of Franklin Delano Roosevelt are permanently part of our archives. Yet the most basic communication in the world—word of mouth—has not progressed, and has even regressed in many areas. A major problem today to mothers (and children) is the so-called "generation gap." More aptly it should be called the communications gap, for the only possible bridge that can span this chasm is verbal communication.

Once children reach the age of sixteen or so, they are influenced very little by parents. Whatever impact a parent wishes to make on the development of the child's personality must be done long before that time. To have a blueprint for the child's life and direct its execution like a marionette show is not now (nor ever was) acceptable. The loving, intuitive parent will try to understand the viewpoints of the child and her motivations and moods. One can lead without force, show by example, and use logical explanation rather than threat of retaliation to accomplish the desired goal.

It is indeeed paradoxical that those parents who oppose sex education in the schools are the ones least qualified to face the problem at home. To be sure, if this group had its way, ignorance of sex would be perpetuated for all time to come. If your answer to a small child who asks where babies come from is the stork, then you yourself are even more in need of sex education than your child! Not only is it a flagrant lie, but it keeps the child in a world of fantasy in which she is already too deeply engrossed. It just makes the world of reality, which brings disappointment and depression to the child, that much harder to face. Furthermore such prevarications cause the child to lose respect for the parent, particularly as a reliable source of information. The door to the communications-generation gap has already started to close.

It is inappropriate, ineffectual, and inexcusable to tell the growing child that sex is dirty, the genital organs unclean and untouchable, and other fantastic unrealities associated with these parts. If it's because you don't know any better, perhaps you should be pitied; but if you are knowledgeable and premeditate such bigotry, then you should be reprimanded. Perhaps in time the child will find out for itself a more truthful perspective, hopefully before you have caused irreparable damage to its future happiness and peace of mind.

Once I had the misfortune to treat a young teen-ager for pregnancy and V.D. I spent about an hour counseling this patient. I told her it was not the end of the world, that her future health, both physically and mentally, should not be affected by her plight, and I suggested that she consider that her period was a little late and we could solve her problem by a simple D. and C. Furthermore I told this girl that sex was a normal expression and that she should feel no guilt or remorse from her experience, that sex is a beautiful experience and under other circumstances could bring her much joy and happiness. Following the D. and C. I gave her prescriptions for the V.D. and birth control pills to avoid similar consequences in the future.

When her mother learned of my suggestion that this girl take birth control pills, she severely chastised me and stated that her daughter had never had intercourse but once in her life and that she had learned her lesson and would never do it again! What a miserable future this poor girl faced. Constant vigilant observation by her mother twenty-four hours a day, repeated rebuking for a vile, debased act, and even suspicious monitoring of her phone calls and letters, not to mention clandestine sneaking to read the girl's diary. Such vitriolic behavior by a mother, as I see it, can only render this child permanently frigid, with a hatred for all men, or lesbian.

Another patient asked me how she should handle her sixteen-year-old daughter's sexual education. I told her that by that age she probably didn't need much in the way of education, but that protection against the perils of pregnancy might be offered at the discretion of the girl. The woman replied, "But Doctor, she is only sixteen. If she were nineteen, I might be more amenable to your suggestion." Then I said, "What do you plan, lady, to give your child some birth control pills on her nineteenth birthday and tell her to go get laid?" As we provide the child with a roof over her head to protect against the elements, as we furnish food to nourish her body, as we provide for her every need, it is also necessary for the loving and sensible parent to protect the young girl against the possibility of pregnancy. As I told this woman, "Lady, you do not have the prerogative of deciding with whom, where or when your daughter first has intercourse, but you do have the prerogative of offering her protec tion."

Although the constant fear of parents is that if they give their children contraceptive advice or pills, this is a "carte blanche" for them to behave promiscuously, my experience would indicate that nothing could be further from the truth! For the most part, the young people who come to me for birth control advice are going steady and have already embarked on the sensuous journey long before they face the mature responsibility of preventing its unfortunate consequences. It is nevertheless true that there are some promiscuous people, but there were some before the pill, there will always be some, and if one thinks the pill is the cause, then the person is either unenlightened, naïve, or dumb. On the other hand, if a girl does happen to be promiscuous, then protection is a necessity!

While we're talking about promiscuity, isn't it diabolical that the most frequent motivation for this type of sexual exploration is lack of parental affection—a search for love unknown at home. In other words, it is not the permissive parent who promulgates promiscuity, but rather the overly protective paragon of propriety who actually predisposes to this form of sexual indiscretion. A constant search for affection and understanding denied by your establishment causes the child to seek artificial pseudo-affection by whatever means seems most accessible at the exigency of the moment, to wit—sex! Before you blame a child for aberrant activity, first analyze yourself. Have you contributed to the problem by your own inadequacy? It is very easy to criticize —particularly a dependent minor—but perhaps if you approached the child with more understanding, she would respond with more maturity!

CHAPTER 19

Youth Without Couth

Our youth now loves luxury. They have bad manners, contempt for authority, and disrespect for older people. Children nowadays are tyrants, they no longer rise when their elders enter the room They contradict their parents, chatter before company, gobble their food, and tyrannize teachers.

——Socrates (Ca. 400 B.C.)

ONE of the basic problems of twentieth-century teen-agers is that their reproductive organs have developed faster than their brains. The current inhabitation of our maternity wards with around 10 percent unmarried women is due to lack of knowledge of contraception, defiance, exhibitionism, or in many instances, just plain stupidity. Despite the abundantly available advice on contraception and the legalization of abortion, many young people refuse to recognize the cause of pregnancy and its prevention. They stick their heads in the sand like an ostrich and feel that this could never happen to them. Too frequently the obstetrician sees them too late for any preventive or interruptive procedure.

Then comes the big internal psychologic conflict—to keep or not to keep the baby. To keep the baby is like a millstone around their necks. They are neither financially able or psychologically attuned to the acceptance of the responsibility of motherhood. Furthermore, few men will consider marrying the mother of an illegitimate child. On the other hand, giving up the baby for adoption causes torn indecision and ambivalence to the mother—the very cause of depression. One never forgets or detaches oneself from the most intense of all human emotions —the maternal instinct. Perhaps in no phase of life is the old adage, "An ounce of prevention is worth a pound of cure," more pertinent!

It is indeed pathetic for me to encounter in my office a sixteen-or seventeen-year-old virgin in request of a premarital examination. By presently available statistics she doesn't have a snowball's chance in hell of a lasting relationship.

As a method of escaping from the establishment, parental authority, and to do one's own thing, the grass always looks greener on the other side of the street. Unfortunately, there is in this instance a gross misinterpretation of sex and love. The teen-age body is capable of sex—in all its forms—but the teen-age mind is incapable of love—everlasting, deep, undying, and unbounded love. The divorce records attest to the accuracy of this statement. Moreover, such marriages seldom endure beyond the expected date of confinement of the first pregnancy, which all too frequently occurs too soon. Then we're back to the plight, almost, of the unwed mother. Only a small legal technicality differentiates between the two.

Just recently I encountered a twenty-three-year-old mother of two who had been divorced three times (her first marriage was at age sixteen). The only comment I could muster was, "Why bother?" There can be little refutation that a three-time loser with two "yard apes" to support is much less nubile than a twenty-three-year-old woman with a modicum of sexual experience. Youth and stupidity go hand in hand but it need not necessarily be so!

ANOREXIA NERVOSA (Voluntary Starvation)

This condition is suffered primarily by teen-age—or sometimes older—girls. Basically it is caused by dietary indiscretion because of the obsessive feeling that one is overweight and that drastic measures must be instituted. The girl goes on a starvation diet, and even after a grossly subnormal weight has been obtained, she continues to diet. By this time the loss of appetite and revulsion to food—even to the point of nausea and vomiting—have occurred. She acquires the figure of a beanpole with droopy or absent breasts, sunken jowls, and spidery legs. She is physically unattractive to everyone except herself for she is still under the misapprehension that the thinner, the more beautiful. Carried to its nth degree, this voluntarily acquired, self-imposed disease can be fatal and *is* in about 10 percent of cases. The victims literally starve themselves to death. Once it has reached the point of no return, even the most heroic medical efforts are of no avail.

On the other end of the spectrum are the teen-agers who overeat to fulfill otherwise not understood emotional needs—low self-esteem, insecurity, parental defiance, fear, and sex. The same factors contribute to other objectionable, nervous habits such as fingernail biting and nose picking.

To be sure, facing growing up in our world today is awe-inspiring with its diverse complexities, competitiveness, and demands. No question, such challenges are depressing and disheartening. It makes youths today reluctant to face this seemingly impregnable bulwark of maturation, accomplishment, and finding their place in society. The overwhelming feeling of insecurity, hopelessness, and despair causes the longing to escape and to forget the world, its responsibilities and obligations.

Unfortunately, too frequently the escape route is paved with drugs and alcohol. Even suicides in young people have reached epidemic proportions. In their fight for flight many young people are inspired by cultists and others who extol the virtues of mind-altering drugs. Since most all of these agents have no medicinal value, the real and long-term pharmacologic effects have never been adequately studied scientifically.

Having been in use for thousands of years, alcohol's effects are well understood—its temporary effect, its predisposition to addiction, and the serious consequences of its abuse.

On the other hand, marijuana has not yet had a full pharmacologic study from the standpoints of immediate and long-term effects. Probably, as with alcohol, occasional *judicious* use of this drug carries minimal risks, but there have been medical reports of permanent brain damage from constant use and over-abuse of this substance.

Hard drugs such as LSD, cocaine, and heroin are *extremely* dangerous and should absolutely be avoided. No physician familiar with emergency room work has failed to encounter the O.D. (overdose) of these agents, the bad, wild trips with LSD, and occasionally unintentional deaths.

Besides the "flashbacks" from LSD and the relatively incurable addiction to cocaine and heroin, the cost of these drugs is high and very few people, especially young people, can afford the "habit." In order to pay for their needs the girls frequently turn to prostitution and the boys to pushing. What an ugly scene! If such an approach is not stifled, then like the spread of a chain letter, the world will eventually become overpopulated with hopheads and harlots.

The world really isn't that bad. Every generation since the beginning of time has had problems to work out. Somehow or other the challenges have been met. Actually the greater the challenge, the greater the opportunity. It should be encouraging to young people today to realize how many things they can do. The future is unbounded for one who perseveres.

In 1870 the head of the United States Patent Office suggested to Congress that the patent office be closed, as everything had already been invented. This was before the invention of the electric light! Today the door is open to anyone with motivation, and not just to those with education. Thomas Edison had only three months of schooling but took out 1,033 patents for his inventions.

CHAPTER 20

Male Ms. Conceptions

IT is difficult for one as knowledgeable as myself to conceive of the ignorance, stupidity, superstitiousness, and general gullibility of many males. It is really no wonder to me that women's lib labels them "male chauvinist pigs." As this book is essentially for women, I am including a few of the common—even ridiculous—male misconceptions so that you may be better informed about these silly notions.

When I was stationed in Japan following World War II the ingenious, enterprising Nipponese capitalized on the popular myth held by many American males that the Oriental vulva is crosswise. They sold pictures galore of Japanese women sitting in sartorial fashion to reveal a resplendent (but obviously artificially retouched) horizontal vulva. The G.I.s bought these pictures in bulk, sent them home to their friends, thus perpetuating this ridiculous concept with pictorial proof!

Another popular, male egocentric misconception is that women when they masturbate use phallic substitutes such as bananas, cucumbers, dildoes or other penis substitutes. As a matter of fact, women rarely use such devices for this purpose. Furthermore the idea that lesbians use phallic symbols or double dildoes for gratification is ridiculous. The last thing a true lesbian is interested in is anything resembling a penis. Nevertheless, the "stag movies" cater to this erroneous concept and thus two purposes are served: more of this kind of movies are sold, and gullible men are furthered in their assurance of the usualness of this form of eroticism. The height of egomania in males is the feeling that if they ever gave a lesbian a good screwing, she would give up her female preference. How stupid can one get!

For some unknown reason, the size of the female breasts presents to some (unsophisticated and unknowledgeable) men an indicator of the woman's sex drive. Actually there is little or no correlation with breast size and sexuality other than the psychological shyness that one occasionally encounters in women who become self-conscious because their breasts are too small (or too large). This concept is held mainly by breast freaks who are really projecting their own proclivities into the personality of others.

Undoubtedly the most common and most erroneous imagery that men hold is that the greatest turn-on is the big penis. Nothing could be further from the truth! As most women with varying sexual experience will attest, the size of the organ is not correlated with their own attainment of orgasm. The skillful, sensuous use of the male appendage is far more important than its size.

Unfortunately, many men are not even aware of the existence of the clitoris, its location, the fact that it is the analog of the penis in the male, and that it is the singular source of orgasm in the female. On the other hand, men are quite knowledgeable in the art of pleasing themselves but refuse to accept the responsibility of satisfying their mates. A most common situation encountered in my office is the woman who comes in with the complaint that something is wrong with *her* because she doesn't have orgasms. My inquiry always is, "Does your mate have orgasms?" When she replies affirmatively, then I say, "Well, you're doing your part, he just isn't doing his." Once a man has an erection, he is immediately ready for intercourse and may expect this unprodigious phenomenon to cause sudden arousal in the woman, such that she can immediately rise to the attainment of instant orgasm to coincide with his premature ejaculation; and he deduces erroneously therefrom that she is frigid or sexually inadequate. Perhaps no better enlightenment on this subject is available than the old saying, "There's no such thing as a frigid woman, only clumsy men." Actually, if you are one of the unfortunate unorgasmic women, your mate needs education, counseling, and indoctrination. In order to help solve *his* problem, first show him your clitoris—tell him that's "where it's at." Masturbate in front of him. Show him what gives you an orgasm. If you are one of the majority of women who needs clitoral stimulation during coitus in addition to penile thrusting, tell him so, and what kind. If you need manual or oral stimulation to arouse your appetite for making love, tell him so. Otherwise you should adopt the Kennedys' football regulation: "If you don't play by my rules, I'll take my ball and go home."

A sensitive, normal man will receive a tremendous ego trip from being able to excite a woman to orgasm, even more so if he can impart to her multiple orgasms—of which most women are capable. On the losing side of the ball game is the man who never brings his female companion to experience her sexually orgasmic potential. He should be avoided like a leper.

The only way to overcome the male Ms. conceptions is by adequate and complete communication in these areas. Tell him like it is, but do it gently! Don't stick a pin in his bubble too fast; it could cause an explosive deflation of the male ego.

CHAPTER 21

The Answer to Cancer

UNQUESTIONABLY the most dreaded disease to all humanity is cancer. It is such a bad word that I have frequently said it should be spelled with four letters!

Although the cause of cancer eludes the knowledge of the most learned and erudite physicians, the Food and Drug Administration has discovered innumerable causes through its unintelligent, unscientific and implausible explanations. We all recall several years ago when the cranberry insecticide was found to be cancer-causing, but more scientific appraisal of the facts indicated that a person would have to eat fifty carloads of cranberries to produce this disease. The most recent breakthrough in the answer to cancer is that chemicals used in the processing of decaffeinated coffee have been shown to be carcinogenic. No doubt the National Cancer Institute will receive a Nobel Prize for this amazing discovery. Other research studies, however, indicate that one would have to drink 50,000,000 cups of decaffeinated coffee daily for an entire lifetime in order to cause cancer—a rather unlikely probability.

The implication of all this is that if one does not smoke, drink decaffeinated coffee, eat cranberries, bacon with sodium nitrite as a preservative, or consume anything colored by Red Dye No. 2, one is thereby forever and forthwith protected against the scourge of cancer! Forget it! It's really not that easy. A disease as prevalent and predatory as cancer will surely require somewhat more sophisticated research to find its cause. As we have conquered the challenge of space, so shall the cause of cancer some day be discovered, but probably not by the F.D.A.

Cancer is the second most common cause of death in the United States, being surpassed only by heart disease. But don't look at this fact with despair. At the turn of the century cancer was virtually 100 percent fatal. Twenty-five years ago only one in four cancers were cured, but today 50 percent of cancers could be cured if all patients were diagnosed and treated in time. Great progress in the treatment of cancer has been made, and unbounded medical research is constantly striving to determine its cause and prevention. Although exact causes are yet to be defined, many related circumstances do offer some insight along this line.

Most cancers are not hereditary, but a woman whose mother or sister has had breast cancer is two to three times more likely to be a victim than one with no familial history of the disease. Furthermore, for one whose mother and sister both have had breast cancer the risk is fifteen times greater. There doesn't seem to be a similar familial trend for other types of cancer.

It is now generally accepted that cigarette smoking increases the incidence of cancer of the lung. Excessive exposure to ultraviolet radiation (sunshine) is associated with cancer of the skin and recent studies report an increased ultraviolet concentration in sunlight, probably due to alterations in the protective ozone layer above the earth. This fact alone would make it unwise for people to voluntarily expose themselves to the sun for the dubious beautification of a tan. Furthermore, sunshine causes dryness and wrinkling of the skin.

Certain types of infections are associated with cancer, but a real causal relationship has yet to be proven. Moreover, there are some noxious and toxic chemicals that are carcinogenic. Chronic irritations, regardless of cause, seem to increase the risk of cancer. Also, we know that certain kinds of cancer attack people of certain age groups and races more frequently.

Although there are many pieces yet missing from the cancer puzzle, there are still many things you can do to at least give the reassurance of doing everything possible to avert death from this dread disease.

Since the discovery of the cytologic smear test for cancer of the uterine cervix by Dr. George H. Papanicolaou in 1943, the deaths from cervical cancer have been drastically reduced and could virtually be eliminated if *all* women would have Pap smears regularly, at least every year and every six months over age thirty-five. Despite the painless simplicity of this test, more than 21,000,000 women in the United States have never had a Pap test. From these 21,000,000 will come the estimated 12,000 deaths that will occur this year from cancer of the cervix.

Since the Pap smear can detect cancer of the cervix from many months to many years before the destructive invasion of the disease occurs, it is at least theoretically possible to find all cases in the very early stage, when virtually 100 percent cure can be effected by surgery.

In anticipation of a Pap test the woman should not douche or use any vaginal medication for several days before the examination; these would remove or alter the vaginal discharge to be examined.

The Pap smear is one of the most reliable and accurate of all medical laboratory tests, but it is only for cancer of the cervix. Any woman over twenty—especially the sexually active—who fails to have this test at least every year is very foolish.

Cancer of the body of the womb only shows up on the Pap smear in only about half the cases. However, cancer of the body of the womb bleeds early; therefore, all women with bleeding (regardless of how slight) between their periods, prolonged menstruation, and particularly bleeding after the menopause need careful evaluation as to the cause of the bleeding, and the alert physician will presume it to be cancer until proven otherwise. If all women with abnormal bleeding sought medical attention immediately, the present cure rate for cancer of the body of the womb of about 75 percent could be increased to over 90 percent.

Most early cancers of the ovary give *no* symptoms. As with most other forms of cancer, pain does *not* occur until the terminal stages. Detection of the cured cases is usually by routine examination. So once again the periodic pelvic checkup is your best bet to avoid disaster.

The treatment of pelvic cancer leaves little or no disfigurement of the body and usually no alteration in sexual functioning other than inability to conceive.

Unquestionably the most feared form of cancer for women is that of the breast. This is due mainly to the disfigurement that follows its surgical treatment. As with all forms of cancer, early detection is our most effective weapon. There are some groups of women who have a higher incidence rate of this disease. They are those with a familial history of breast cancer, those with previous cancer of one breast, those who have had no pregnancies or whose first pregnancy occurred after age twenty-five, and those women who reach menopause after the age of fifty. Birth control pills and other hormones are not a causal factor in this disease. The "old wives' tale" that injury such as a single blow to the breast can cause cancer has never been medically proven. It's just that many women first notice a lump in the breast after such an injury because the injury attracts their attention to the breast. Then they feel a tumor that has been there but has not been noticed before this time.

All women panic when they find a lump in the breast, but actually only about one out of five is cancer. However, some benign tumors can become malignant if neglected. Although we think of breast cancer as a disease of middle-aged and older women, its incidence is not entirely limited to any age group.

Cancer of the breast is curable and with early detection the cure rate approaches 90 percent. Despite the advent of complicated and sophisticated diagnostic techniques such as mammography, xerography, and thermography, 90 percent of cases of breast cancer are first found by the women themselves. Monthly self-examination is still the best and most effective method of early detection of breast cancer.

For the menstruating woman, the self-examination should be performed at the end of a day or two after the period because the hormones that control menstruation also affect the glandular tissues of the breast. Before the period, sometimes there is cystic enlargement of the breast glands that simulates the feel of a bag of jellybeans. Often a woman will confuse these normal changes and run to the doctor immediately, only to be told, "Come back after your period for a recheck."

If you are postmenopausal, check your breasts on a regular monthly basis. If you are taking cyclic hormones, the examination should be made on the day you restart your hormone pills (or take your shot).

In order to effectively examine your breasts, first stand in front of a mirror in a well-lighted room with your arms relaxed at your sides and look for any difference in the size and shape of the breast and nipples. Look for any retraction of the nipple or dents in the skin, ulcerations or sores of the skin, or an orange-peel texture of the skin. Then raise your arms overhead and look for the same signs or any difference in the breasts from the arm-down position. Next, place both hands on your hips and squeeze inward, thus contracting the muscles under the breasts. Once again, look for the same changes outlined above.

Next, lie down on a firm bed or couch. If your breasts are large, place a small pillow or folded towel under the shoulder of the side being examined. To examine your right breast, place your right hand behind your head and your left hand flatly on the breast, first feeling the nipple, then gradually going around and around the nipple area in concentric circles until all of the breast has been felt. Gently squeeze the nipple to see if there is any discharge. Reverse the procedure for the left breast.

Usually cancer of the breast is a stony-hard lump, not tender, irregular in shape, and not freely movable. However, any lump or areas of tenderness, and particularly any change in your breast since the previous examination should be reported without delay to the doctor.

Unfortunately, too many women feel that self-examination and manipulation of the breast is base, lewd, and immoral—a form of masturbation. As has been pointed out, today this is a woman's best chance to escape death from this cause. When you fail or refuse to check your own breasts, you bet your life!

Since the recent affliction of both Betty Ford and Happy Rockefeller with cancer of the breast, there has been an acute awareness of all women as to the frequency and seriousness of this disease. As in all situations of panic, there is always associated some overreaction. Women who have never checked their own breasts and have not had an examination for five or ten years are flocking to the doctors' offices for breast checks. Imaginary pains and lumps are now being found in epidemic proportions. Many women insist upon X-ray mammography, xerography, or thermography without the least idea of the indications, contraindications, and limitations of these procedures. Furthermore, any form of examination today does not rule out the occurrence of cancer tomorrow! Sometimes these examinations give a false sense of security to the point that the most important detection tool we now have—periodic self-examination—is neglected!

MAMMOGRAPHY

This is a soft-tissue X-ray examination of the breast which has been helpful in the diagnosis of cancer of the breast. Although it is possible to detect cancer of the breast by this technique, when no palpable lump is present the chances of any one woman at any one time finding an otherwise unsuspected cancer by this technique is extremely remote. Moreover, the use of this procedure for periodic examinations—say every six months—is both economically unreasonable and physically unfeasible because of the presently limited facilities for such examinations. Also the accuracy of the interpretations of mammograms is dependent upon the ability and skill of the radiologist.

The Food and Drug Advisory Committee has recently recommended that mammography should not be used routinely in women under the age of thirty-five who have no complaint, no personal or strong familial history of cancer, and no physical evidence of cancer. It is ridiculous for young women to submit themselves to the yet unknown hazards of the biologic effects of repeated low-dosage radiation (which is cumulative over one's entire life span) without reason. To be sure, mammography is an important contribution to the early diagnosis of cancer of the breast and the differential diagnosis of cancer and other benign diseases, but let your doctor decide when and if you need it.

XEROGRAPHY

This is merely a variation of mammography which electronically prints the image on paper instead of film. It requires less radiation exposure, but in general its limitations and advantages are the same as film mammography.

THERMOGRAPHY

This is a procedure which detects changes in heat transmitted into a photographic image. Many breast conditions—both benign and malignant—are associated with increased heat. Thermography is not then an indicator of cancer as such. It is a useful, diagnostic tool, but it can be overused and erroneously interpreted. Once again, let the doctor decide.

Those women who do have to face the problem or possibility of cancer of the breast react with despair, resentment, anger, and pathos. The fear of pain, disfigurement, mutilation, the unknown—even death—distorts their sense of reason. The fear of rejection by one's mate for the loss of part of her body, particularly one of sensuous significance, is alarming.

For the most part, these fears are unfounded or, at least, considerably exaggerated, for as pointed out above, most breast cancers are curable and most men accept the confrontation with this problem with compassionate understanding.

The surgical treatment of cancer of the breast depends on the extent of the disease, the skill and training of the attending surgeon, and many other factors. At present, confirmatory diagnosis by frozen section at the operating table followed by radical mastectomy (removal of the entire breast, the underlying muscles, and lymph glands in the armpits) is the most usual; however, excellent and comparable results may be obtained with the less mutilating (and functionally less impairing of the arm movements) simple mastectomy—removal of only the breast itself—followed by radiation or chemical therapy.

Perhaps it would be more appropriate for those women who find an early cancer to look upon this as a blessing rather than a calamity, for with proper treatment most of them can enjoy long, fruitful, and fulfilling lives.

Having attended many cases of terminal cancer, I have always been impressed with the hopeful outlook of these patients and their continuing confidence for their recovery. The initial fears are replaced by the will to live or—at worst—acceptance of the inevitable.

Of the less frequent cancers of the body, many of the cardinal signs are too often ignored, such as presuming that rectal bleeding is due to hemorrhoids—it may be the first sign of cancer of the bowel. Never take for granted that a persistent cough is a cigarette cough or cold—it may be cancer of the lung.

Do not ignore growth, bleeding, or enlargement of a mole—particularly the black ones with hairs growing in them—these signs could herald malignant change. In general, constant vigilance and regular checkups are our best known ways today to conquer cancer.

The warning signals of cancer as specified by the American Cancer Society are:

1. Unusual bleeding or discharge
2. A lump or thickening in the breast or elsewhere
3. A sore that does not heal
4. Change in bowel or bladder habits
5. Hoarseness or cough
6. Indigestion or difficulty in swallowing
7. Change in size or color of a wart or mole

To ignore any of these signs is like coming to a railroad crossing when the red light is flashing and you go on anyway, not believing that a train is really coming. Not heeding these signals could cause your death from stupidity, coincidentally complicated by cancer!

CHAPTER 22

Twilight Time

UNFORTUNATELY, most women look upon the so-called "change of life" with awe, fear, and trepidation. Lack of knowledge and understanding of this important phase of living and old wives' tales contribute in large measure to this apprehension. Even the term "change of life" implies a drastic transfiguration such as occurs in *Dr. Jekyll and Mr. Hyde,* and the term "climacteric" implies a critical period of culmination to be followed only by a downhill course. For this reason I prefer the more appropriate and correct term—menopause.

Really, one should look upon the menopause as the pause that refreshes, for one no longer need fear the possibility of pregnancy—an event generally most undesirable in women over forty. Also, by this time one's children are usually grown, married, or gone, and some degree of financial security has been obtained. It would seem more appropriate to consider the menopause as the time of fulfillment.

From a physiologic standpoint, the only change that occurs

is the cessation of the function of the ovaries. No longer are eggs produced—who wants them at this time?—and the output of the female hormone, estrogen, wanes. If one considers that girls before the beginning of menstruation had no significant amount of estrogen, and they were not miserable, depressed and unhappy, there is no reason for them to be so after the withdrawal of this hormone.

Although the menopause usually begins during the late forties, rare instances occur as early as thirty and as late as sixty. Some women experience no signs of the menopause, other than the cessation of menstruation, but most women do have some physical and psychologic symptoms, which may vary tremendously from woman to woman.

The most common physical symptom is hot flashes. These are often described as like heat waves rising in the upper body and head. In some women this may be only a mild warming sensation, while others may have a severe feeling of intense heat associated with perspiration, followed by chills. These may occur every several days or even several times a day, and are more frequent in the summer months. Although the exact cause of the dilation of the blood vessels producing hot flashes is not known, it is obviously related to estrogen withdrawal because replacement of this hormone will usually stop them.

Other physical symptoms may include sagging of the breasts, dryness and wrinkling of the skin, numbness and crawling sensations of the skin, muscular aches and pains, and headaches. However, graying of the hair and the occasional growth of hair on the face are *not* due to estrogen withdrawal, though the texture of the hair may be affected. One definite change that is directly related to hormonal deficiency is atrophic (senile) vaginitis—a thinning of the lining tissues of the vagina causing soreness, dryness, and discharge. There is usually associated loss of elasticity of the vaginal and surrounding tissues. This gives rise to pain on intercourse and sometimes loss of bladder control.

The psychologic symptoms of the menopause are more varied and more difficult to define. Many women nearing or over forty use the excuse of "change of life" to explain away any emotional or nervous problem they might have. Also many of the psychologic symptoms associated with the menopause are merely exaggerations of previously present psychological predilections. Nervous spells, irritability, unfounded fears, insomnia, crying spells, feeling blue or depressed, and other mood changes are frequently encountered at this time. Other symptoms which are probably more psychologic than physiologic are dizziness, lapse of memory, palpitations of the heart, constipation, diarrhea, nausea, fatigue, and also the tendency to put on weight. The menopause does *not*, as the "old wives" say, cause a woman to "lose her mind."

Many women think that the menopause marks the end of their sexual urges and performance potential. This is totally untrue. Actually, estrogen has little or no effect on the sex drive of women. The relief from the fear of pregnancy—both to the woman and her husband—coupled with the fear that time is running out usually causes a rejuvenation and intensification of sexual activity. Furthermore, just as experience in the kitchen makes one a better cook, by this time (if the marriage is still flourishing) bedroom compatibility has probably reached a high peak. As a matter of fact, continued active sex life after the menopause is quite healthy for women (and men) from both a physical and psychological standpoint. It is truly unfortunate that despite available information regarding the menopause, the myths concerning it are so ingrained in our society that that they all too frequently surpass one's ability to reason. Usually women become depressed at this time because they fear their loss of femininity, their loss of sensual appeal to the opposite sex, and the fact that they are growing old. Actually these fears are more fantasy than fact. Some of the sexiest, most alluring women I have ever known were postmenopausal.

The cessation of menstruation does not often occur abruptly, but rather occasional or frequent missed periods is the usual pattern. Most women panic at this point for the fear of pregnancy. Although pregnancies are rather rare at this time, contraception should be continued until one has been six to twelve months without a period. Once again the gossip-mongering, spiteful, fear-provoking "old wives" have assured every maturing woman of the increased fertility that occurs near the menopause as a pen that flows more freely just before it becomes dry. They all know of innumerable women who became pregnant at this time. Isn't it amazing that obstetricians haven't seen them? They must have given birth at home by midwives!

One point that I cannot stress too much is that bleeding between the periods is *never* normal. Too many women have been told that all kinds of bleeding can occur *normally* with the menopause. As a case in point, a forty-five-year-old woman from a rural area had experienced bleeding off and on for six months. Her "friends" assured her that "everyone" had this at her age and that she need not see a doctor. When I examined her I found a very far advanced, hopeless cancer of the womb, beyond medical help. Her "friends" began to dig her grave with their misinformed, unknowledgeable admonition. Don't ever bet your life on free advice! Bleeding between the periods or excessive or prolonged bleeding with the periods may be a sign of serious disease. See your doctor; don't ask a friend.

Another problem women face in the postmenopausal period is osteoporosis—a disease characterized by thinning of the bones, and shortening and stooping of the stature results. As many as one out of four women may have this condition to a greater or lesser degree. Surely you have seen the bent-over old ladies severely afflicted with this condition. Fortunately, it can almost always be prevented by the administration of hormones.

Although not a panacea, the administration of the female hormone, estrogen, is to date the closest thing we have to the

Fountain of Youth. Ponce de Leon would have truly been proud if he had discovered this substance. Estrogen relieves most of the physical and many of the psychological changes of the menopause. In addition to preventing osteoporosis, it helps maintain the tone of the skin and the texture of the hair. It will completely relieve atrophic vaginitis, and there is some evidence to suggest that it reduces the incidence of heart attacks.

Nevertheless there has been a recent barrage by the F.D.A. that estrogens administered after the menopause may cause an increased incidence of cancer of the body of the womb. These reports have not been substantiated and, as a matter of fact, have even been refuted in many articles in medical journals. This controversy is not new: when I was a student thirty-odd years ago the question of whether or not estrogens caused uterine cancer was popular. Although the dilemma has not yet been solved, neither has its converse. My wife of twenty-five years takes estrogens.

Despite the multiple advantages of estrogen, there are some contraindications to its use; therefore have a thorough checkup by a competent physician before embarking on its use. Furthermore, this is a potent hormone drug, and regular examinations (at least every six months) should be had during its use. Today most gynecologists will agree that the advantages of estrogen in postmenopausal women far outweigh any of its possible disadvantages, but it should always be taken under a doctor's close supervision.

Some women realize even better results in the treatment of their menopausal troubles with a mixture of estrogen and testosterone (male hormone). The effect of testosterone in women essentially enhances their feeling of well-being, and a few also experienced an increase in libido. On the other hand, excessive dosage with this hormone can cause growth of hair on the face, deepening of the voice, and enlargement of the clitoris. As with most aspects of medical treatment, judicious judgment must be used in planning a program of treatment of the menopause.

When the menopause is produced surgically by removal of the ovaries, the signs and symptoms are the same as with the natural menopause, but they occur more abruptly. Many women have the mistaken notion that the removal of the womb (hysterectomy) causes menopause. The womb secretes no hormones nor rids the body of any toxic substances. Removal of only the womb does cause a cessation of menstruation which, after all, is merely a response to the hormones of the ovary, and pregnancy is no longer possible. Otherwise, hysterectomy makes *no* change in a woman, physiologically, psychologically, or sexually, unless she has been brainwashed before and after this operation into believing such rot as that this makes one an incomplete woman, that she will never be able to function normally sexually, that she will lose her mind, and that she will gain weight. This is all 100 percent bunkum.

The treatment of the surgical menopause is the same as the natural menopause, unless contraindicated by such diseases as cancer or endometriosis.

The menopause is not the end of the world—it merely heralds a new stage of life, the stage of maturity, fulfillment, and enrichment. If you can accept the normal maturing stage of life beginning with the menopause with insight and understanding, then you are best endowed to live happily ever after.

Glossary

Abortion The expulsion of a fetus from the womb before it is viable. A miscarriage, usually by artificial or surgical methods.

Abscess A swollen, inflamed area in body tissues in which pus gathers.

Allergic Hypersensitivity to a drug, food, pollen, wool, etc., causing a bodily reaction.

Amenorrhoea Absence or abnormal stoppage of menstruation.

Amniocentesis Procedure wherein a needle is passed through the abdominal wall of pregnant woman into womb, withdrawing some of the amniotic fluid to determine sex of child and/or whether fetus is defective.

Amniotic Fluid A thin, watery, serum-like fluid in which the fetus is immersed.

Anal Erotism Sexual stimulation of the anus.

Anal Intercourse Intercourse or copulation in which the penis is inserted into the anus.

Anal Sphincter There are two sphincters (muscles) in the anus. One external extending from the coccyx to the perineum, the other an internal circular muscle in the rectum.

Anilingus Oral manipulation of the anus for sexual stimulation.

Anorexia Nervosa Voluntary starvation. A nervous disorder causing loss of appetite and revulsion to food. Obsessive desire to be thin.

Antibiotic Therapy Use of antibiotics; a chemical substance produced by microorganisms which has the capacity in dilute solution to inhibit growth of or destroy bacteria.

Antiseptic Disinfectant, germicide. A substance that prevents or arrests the growth or action of microorganisms either by inhibiting their activity or destroying them.

ANUS External opening from the bowel.

ANXIETY NEUROSIS A chronic state of apprehension, uncertainty and fear.

APHRODISIAC DIET Foods that are supposed to be, or rumored to be, sexually stimulating.

ARTIFICIAL BREASTS Breasts created by implants of silicone or other plastic substances; or a synthetic false breast or bra insert worn by women having had a mastectomy.

ASYMPTOMATIC Showing or causing no symptoms.

ATROPHY Shrinkage and drying up as in old age. Sometimes during menopause, when there is an imbalance of hormones, women suffer vaginal atrophy, a thinning of the lining tissues of the vagina causing soreness, dryness and discharge.

BACTERIAL FLORA Bacterial plant life of a given area, such as the bacterial content of the intestinal canal.

BACTERIAL VAGINITIS A bacterial infection. Produces foul, greyish, non-irritating discharge. Simultaneous treatment of sexual contacts essential to prevent reinfection.

BACTERIOCIDAL An antibacterial antibody which causes death of the bacteria.

BARTHOLIN GLANDS Two small reddish-yellow bulbs, one on either side of the vaginal opening.

BASAL THERMOMETER Thermometer for measuring cellular activity by the rate of heat given off after a 12-hour rest and fast. Used to determine fertile time in women's cycle.

BLADDER Membranous sac situated in the anterior part of the pelvic cavity which serves as a reservoir for the urine.

BULBOCAVERNOSUS Central point of perineum; constricts, contracts urethra.

CAESAREAN SECTION Delivery of the fetus by an incision through the abdominal and uterine wall.

CANDIDA ALBICANS Fungus infection of the vagina.

CANTHARIDES (*Spanish Fly*) An aphrodisiac.

CARCINOGENIC Having properties which produce cancer.

CERVIX The neck of the womb, the part that extends into the vagina.

CHANCRE A hard ulcer, ¼″ to ¾″ in diameter, usually singular and not tender, a primary lesion of syphilis.

CHANCROID Soft chancre infection of the genitals, caused by specific bacterium, the Hemophilus Ducreyi.

CHLOASMA Brownish area of discoloration of the skin—particularly forehead and face.

CIRCULATION Movement of the blood in the veins and arteries throughout the body.

CIRRHOSIS Chronic inflammation of area between cells of any organ. Marked by progressive destruction of cells and increase of conncctive tissue.

CLITORIS A small, elongated, erectile body, situated at the front angle of the vulva. Homologue of the penis in the male.
COCAINE A local narcotic anesthetic.
COCCYX Tail bone.
COITUS Sexual intercourse.
COLON The part of the large intestine extending to the rectum.
COLOSTOMY Opening the bowel through abdominal wall.
CONDOM A covering for the penis, used to prevent pregnancy and venereal disease.
CONDYLOMATA ACUMINATA (Venereal warts) Viral infection of venereal spread. Hormonal changes of pregnancy sometimes cause these warts. Found in ano-genital area.
CONJUGAL Pertaining to sexual intercourse.
CONTRACEPTION Anything or any effort used to prevent pregnancy.
CONTRAINDICATION Any condition, especially any condition of disease which renders some particular line of treatment improper or undesirable.
COWPER'S GLANDS Glands in man's groin which create pre-ejaculatory secretion.
CUNNILINGUS Oral stimulation of the vulva.
CYST A sac internal or external, normal or otherwise, which contains a liquid or semisolid substance.
CYSTITIS Infection of the bladder.
CYSTOCELE Herniation or protrusion of the bladder into the vagina.
CYTOLOGIC SMEAR TEST (pap test) Test for cancer of the uterine cervix using a smear of uterine secretion.
D&C Scraping of the lining of the womb; used in cases of miscarriage and abortion.
DIAPHRAGM Rubber disc used with spermacide jelly inserted into vagina covering cervix; for contraceptive purposes.
DIETHYLSTILBESTEROL A compound used in treating menopausal symptoms, vaginitis and suppressing lactation.
DILATIONS The action of stretching or enlarging an opening or canal, as in childbirth the uterus must dilate to allow passage of the fetus.
DOUCHE Internal irrigation of the vagina.
DYSENTERY Inflammation of the intestines, especially of the colon, and accompanied by pain in the abdomen and acute diarrhea.
DYSPAREUNIA Difficult or painful coitus in women.
EJACULATION A sudden expulsion of semen at the climax of sexual activity in the male.
ENDOMETRIOSIS A condition in which tissue resembling the uterine mucous membrane occurs in various locations in the pelvic cavity.
ENDOMETRIUM Mucous membrane that lines the cavity of the uterus.
ERECTION Fullness and firmness of the penis or clitoris from sexual excitement, due to engorgement of these organs with blood.
EROGENOUS ZONES Areas of the body that produce erotic feelings.
EROTIC Pertaining to love or lust.

ESCHERICHIA COLI Organisms found in lower bowel, usually non-pathogenic.
ESTROGEN The female hormone produced by the ovary.
FALLOPIAN TUBE The tube connecting the womb to the ovary, through which the sperm and the egg unite to cause pregnancy.
FELLATIO The act of stimulation of the penis with the mouth.
FERTILIZATION The fusion of a spermatazoon with an ovum.
FETISHES Any non-sexual object that excites erotic feeling, such as a glove or a shoe.
FETUS An unborn child.
FIBROIDS Benign tumors of the uterus, made up of uterine muscle tissue.
FLACCIDITY Weak, lax or soft, as in a limp or non-erect penis, or a muscularly weak vagina.
FLAGELLATION Whipping. Can be a source of erotic pleasure.
FRIGIDITY Sexual coldness or indifference in the female.
GENITALIA The reproductive organs.
GERMAN MEASLES An incubatory disease which produces fever, sore throat and a rash. Particularly dangerous to women in early months of pregnancy because of possible damage to the fetus.
GONORRHEA (*clap*) A contagious, catarrhal inflammation of the genital mucous membrane, transmitted chiefly by intercourse. Symptoms—pain, difficulty in urinating and a foul, mucous discharge.
GRANULOMA INGUINALE Venereal infection, causing lesions on vulva, vagina and enlarged inguinal lymph nodes that can ulcerate and cause extensive destruction.
GYNECOLOGY Branch of medicine which treats disease of the genital tract in women.
HEMORRHOID A pile; an enlarged and tortuous vein, artery or lymph vessel in the rectum.
HERNIATION The abnormal protrusion of an organ or other body structure through a defect in a covering membrane, muscle or bone.
HEROIN A habit-forming pain reliever and sedative.
HERPES VIRUS DISEASE Type 1. Occurs above the waist, typical fever blister. Type 2. Occurs in genital region, blistery lesion.
HYMEN A fold of mucous membrane found in virgins which partially blocks the entrance to the vagina. Also called the "maidenhead."
HYPERHIDROSIS Excessive sweating.
HYSTERECTOMY Surgical removal of the womb. A total hysterectomy is a removal of the entire womb, including cervix. Sub-total hysterectomy is a removal of the body of the womb, leaving cervix.
IMPOTENCE Lack of sexual response or failure to achieve erection in males.
INCUBATION The period between implanting of an infectious disease and the appearance of symptoms.
INFECTION Invasion of the body by disease-producing microorganisms and the reaction of the tissue to their presence and to the toxins generated by them.

INFERTILITY Barren or sterile; unable to reproduce.
INTERCOURSE Sexual copulation.
INTRAUTERINE Device (I.U.D.) Polyester plastic device inserted into uterus for contraceptive purposes.
LABIA MAJORA Outer folds of skin of vulva, lip shaped, covered with hair.
LABIA MINORA Inner lips of vulva, having no hair and more erogenous than labia majora.
LACTATION Secretion of milk from breast, as in period of nursing.
LACTOBACILLUS ACIDOPHILUS A bacterial inhabitant of the normal bowel, especially numerous in infants and adults on a high-milk or carbohydrate diet.
LACTOBACILLUS EODERLEINS Normal bacteria occurring in vaginal secretion.
LATENT Lying hidden and undeveloped within a person.
LEVATOR ANI Muscle that draws anus upward, forward, and supports internal organs.
LIBIDO Sexual drive.
LIGAMENT Band of tough tissue connecting bone or holding organs in place.
MAMMOGRAPHY Soft tissue examination of the breast, using radiation photography.
MASOCHISM Getting sexual pleasure from being dominated, mistreated or hurt physically by one's partner.
MASTECTOMY Surgical removal of the breast.
MENOPAUSE End of reproductive era, menstruation, but not of sexual appreciation.
MENSTRUATION Regular, usually monthly, discharge of blood from the womb, beginning at puberty and ending at menopause.
METABOLISM The sum of all the physical and chemical processes by which the human body is maintained.
MICROORGANISM A minute living organism, too small to see without a microscope.
MOLLUSCUM CONTAGIOSUM Virus disease marked by round skin bubbles, containing semi-solid fluid, usually appearing on face.
MONS VENERIS A rounded prominence at the pubis of a woman.
NECROSIS Death of a cell or a group of cells that are in contact with living tissue.
NEISSERIA GONORRHEA A parasitic form of gonorrhea.
ORGASM The climax or culmination of a sexual act.
OSTEOPOROSIS Disease characterized by thinning of the bones and shortening and stooping of stature. Usually post-menopause.
OVARY Female sex gland, counterpart of the testicle in the male; produces eggs and female hormones.
OVULATION Process by which the ovary discharges the egg.
OVUM Female egg.
PATHOLOGIC Diseased.

PEDICULOSIS PUBIS (crabs, lice) Infestation of little animals usually found in pubic hair; causes itching.

PENDULOUS Extremely large, hanging loosely (describing breasts).

PENIS Male sexual appendage. Erectile organ with which he has intercourse.

PERINEAL EXERCISE Strengthening sphincter or tightening muscle to bladder by doing contractions that cut off urine mid-stream.

"THE PILL" Combination of estrogen and progesterone, taken during menstrual cycle to prevent the fertilization of the ovum. A contraceptive device.

PLACENTA Membrane filament through which nutritive supplies pass to fetus.

PODOPHYLLIN Chemical treatment for genital warts.

POTENCY Sexual prowess; also relates to one's ability to reproduce.

PROCTOLOGIC Pertaining to the rectum and anus.

PROGESTERONE A female hormone produced by the ovary after the egg is released.

PROLAPSE OF THE UTERUS Falling or droppage of the womb.

PROPHYLACTIC A remedy which tends to ward off disease.

PROSTATE GLAND Gland in men which surrounds the neck of the bladder and urethra; in older men sometimes becomes diseased (prostatitis) and has to be removed.

PROSTHESIS Replacement of a bodily part, such as eye, leg, tooth by an artificial one.

PRURITUS VULVAE A vaginal infection causing burning, itching irritation.

PSYCHOEGOPATH One who is really crazy about one's self.

PSYCHOLOGIC Physical manifestations due to nervous or mental causes.

PSYCHOSEMENALYSIS The psychologic reaction to semen and its contents.

PUBERTY Time of sexual development in young people.

PUBIC BONE The front of the pelvic bone at the bottom of the abdomen.

PUBOCOCCYGEUS Sphincter contracter of lower vagina which passes from back of pubic bone to tail bone. Some of its fibers blend with urethral and vaginal walls and surround the anus.

PULMONARY EMBOLISM Blood clots in the lungs.

PYORRHEA A discharge of pus.

RECTOCELE Herniation or protrusion of the rectum into the vagina.

RECTUM Lower portion of the large bowel, just above the anus.

RETROGRADE MENSTRUATION Going back to menstruation, as sometimes happens during menopause, or when menstruation has ceased due to birth control pills and then returns.

RHYTHM (safe period) Intercourse based on timing to avoid event of ovulation.

SEMEN Fluid the male ejaculates which carries sperm cells.

SILICONE IMPLANTS Plastic encased silicone bags surgically placed in the breasts, to enlarge them.

SPERM The male seed, which causes pregnancy.

SPERMICIDES (VAGINAL) Form of contraception, creams, jels, suppositories and foam supposed to kill sperm on contact.

SPHINCTER A muscle used for opening and closing, such as the anal sphincter.

STRESS INCONTINENCE OF URINE Loss of urinary control.

STRIAE GRAVIDARUM Reddish brown, later lighter stripes that occur on the abdomen during pregnancy called stretch marks.

SUPERFETATION Conception during an existing pregnancy. Cannot happen in humans.

SYNDROME A group of symptoms of a particular disease.

SYPHILIS A venereal disease—primary lesion, chancre-hard, usually singular and not tender; secondary symptom, generalized red raised skin rash frequently covering whole body. Highly contagious.

TESTOSTERONE A male hormone.

THERMOGRAPHY A procedure that detects changes in heat in breast, transmits into photographic image. Used to detect disease.

THROMBOPHLEBITIS Blood clot in veins of legs.

THROMBOSIS Blood clot.

TRANSVESTITE Someone who likes to "dress up" in clothes of the opposite sex.

TREPONEMA PALLIDUM Corkscrew-shaped organism, caused by syphilis; crosses afterbirth into body of fetus.

TRICHOMONAS VAGINITIS Not venereal disease but transmitted sexually. Causes foul vaginal discharge, itching and ulceration of vulva and vagina. Cause: a small one-celled parasitic animal.

TUBAL LIGATION Surgical sterilization of female, by tying or cutting off of the fallopian tubes.

URETHRITIS Inflammation of the urethra or tube from the bladder to the outside of the vagina.

UTERINE MYOMAS Fibroids.

UTERUS The womb. It menstruates as a reflection of the function of the ovaries and is the carrier of the fetus, but has no sexual function.

VAGINA Birth canal or opening from vulva to the womb.

VASECTOMY Surgical sterilization of the male. Tubes carrying the sperm are ligated so that no sperm cells occur in ejaculation. This does not otherwise interfere with male sexual enjoyment.

VENA CAVA The venous trunk for the lower extremities and for the pelvic and abdominal organs.

VULVA The external female genitalia.

VULVITIS Inflammation of the vulva.

VULVOVAGINITIS Inflammation of the vulva and vagina at the same time.

WOMB See UTERUS.

XEROGRAPHY Electronically prints on paper the image of the breast, using low radiation. Used to detect cancer or pre-cancerous conditions.